HELP YOUR CHILD LOSE WEIGHT AND KEEP IT OFF

HELP YOUR CHILD LOSE WEIGHT AND KEEP IT OFF

BY GUSSIE MASON

Published in association with
Parade Magazine

GROSSET & DUNLAP
Publishers New York

Published Simultaneously in Canada
Library of Congress catalog card number: 74-18874
ISBN: 0-448-02160-9

First Printing
Printed in the United States of America

Contents

HELP YOUR CHILD LOSE WEIGHT AND KEEP IT OFF

1

Beginning with Basics

Let's talk plainly. Your child is fat and you would like to help your child lose weight. Well, I can help you.

By now, of course, you've probably tried crash diets, special diets, medical diets, everything but the drinking man's diet. They all worked for a short time, but then something happened —somehow all those pounds your child thought were gone forever came sneaking back.

Diets are doomed from the start because they never get at the heart of the problem; they never change a child's basic eating patterns. Once the dieter has lost as much weight as he wants, he starts slipping back into his old eating habits and pretty soon he is as heavy as he was before.

The system I now use at my two camps grew out of my own painful experiences with being overweight. For almost a generation, I have been helping girls at Camp Stanley and boys at Camp Tahoe lose as much as 40 pounds during an eight-week summer stay. And to have more fun than they ever thought possible for "fat people."

Naturally, you won't be able to duplicate the completely controlled environment I can create at camp. But you will enjoy advantages that I don't have. Your child won't have to adjust to a new environment and new people. Your child will have the help and support of your whole family when he or she makes up his mind to lose weight.

Losing weight is a physical process, but never underestimate the power of love and understanding from parents, brothers, and sisters. Without the support of one's family, I believe that no child can hope to lose weight and keep it off.

The place to start helping your child lose weight is the doctor's office. The chances are only one out of a hundred that there is a firm medical reason why your child is overweight, but you must still allow for the possibility. You should have your doctor check for latent diseases such as diabetes that might be activated by a sudden change in your child's eating habits.

Even if there is no medical reason for your child's overweight condition and no possibility of a diet triggering medical problems, you may still find your doctor reluctant to allow your child to diet until he has passed puberty. Does this mean you can do nothing to help your overweight child until he is a teen-ager?

Not at all! At the very least, by following some of the suggestions in this book, you can keep your child from gaining *more* weight. Simple tricks such as cutting down the size of his portions and stocking up on fruit to replace candies and sweets can work wonders.

But let's assume that there is no medical reason for your child to be fat, and your doctor thinks it would be a fine idea if you could help him lose weight. You must then begin to analyze your child's world in order to discover why he has put on so much weight.

Overeating is really a collection of bad habits. Before you can help your child develop new habits, you must try to understand why he developed the old ones. How often has your child complained of being "starved?" Even though he looks like he has been eating too much for years, he may indeed be undernourished from the viewpoint of proper nutrition. The person who has the habit of devouring junk foods that give him a quick burst of energy and then burn out quickly often finds himself feeling famished. For instance, a slice of layer cake and a hamburger patty contain the same number of calories. But the layer cake releases its calories quickly into the blood stream and once they are burned up, the person feels hungry again. The meat patty, on the other hand, releases its calories slowly, giving the person a steady flow of energy.

Scientifically speaking, a calorie is the amount of heat needed to raise the temperature of one gram of water one degree centigrade. To the body, a calorie is a measure of the amount of energy that is produced when the body burns food. If we take in more calories than we need, if we eat food that produces bursts of energy rather than a steady flow, or if we fail to use up the number of calories we produce by activity and exercise, we get fat.

Remember Ivan Pavlov's famous experiment with the dogs? Whenever the Russian scientist rang a bell, the dogs would salivate as though they were hungry. They would exhibit all the signs of being famished, although they had just eaten.

Appetite in human beings functions the same way. It's a product of conditioning. Certain things will stimulate our salivary glands into activity and we will think we are hungry, although our bodies have already consumed all the food we need to produce our daily quota of energy.

Before you can change your child's eating habits, you must understand what formed his appetite.

1. ***Did the baby fat never go away?***

Relatives applaud a chubby, rosy-cheeked baby. So some mothers continue feeding the child too much, unconsciously trying to keep their child healthy looking. Other mothers use food as an emotional support. When the baby cries for love, the mother soothes him with a warm bottle. The baby learns to accept the bottle as a substitute mother. When the child later runs into the emotional troubles that all children encounter, he turns naturally to the solace of food. And he gets fat.

2. ***Is your household routine irregular?***

Mother is running off to a meeting, Dad is working late at the office, sister has been talking to her boyfriend since three in the afternoon, brother is at football practice. Somehow in the midst of all these activities, the fat child is supposed to not only make sure he gets fed—or more often, feed himself—but also to keep track of his diet.

On an eat-and-run schedule, it's almost impossible for a mature adult to control his weight. It *is* an impossible job to ask a child to do.

3. ***Does your child come from a fat environment?***

There are some facts that are hard to look squarely in the eye. But if parents expect their children to be realistic about weight control, they had better start by being realistic about themselves. Fewer than 10 percent of the children of normal-weight parents are fat. When one parent is fat, the chances are two in five that the child will be fat. When both parents are fat, the chances are four in five that they will have fat children. That means there is an 80 percent chance that fat parents will have fat children.

If overweight parents want to help their overweight child to reduce, they must be ready to change some of their eating habits, too.

4. ***Did your child learn bad eating habits at an early age?***

The Jewish mother who prepares knishes and blintzes, the Puerto Rican mother who whips up a plate of rice and beans, the second-generation Italian mother who weighs down the table with big plates of pasta are all looking after their families as good mothers should. Unfortunately, they are unconsciously teaching their children to be fat.

I am not saying that children have to forget their cultural heritage and eat nothing but bland, colorless foods. But mothers have to be willing to learn new ways to cook traditional dishes if they want to help slim down their children.

5. ***Has the home life changed dramatically?***

When a child moves from city to city, as military families do so often, it is often difficult for the youngster to settle down, meet new friends, and find new activities. During this period, physical activity drops, and there is often an increase in weight.

Moreover, many children who have learned to soothe their emotions with food, eat more because they are feeling upset by all the changes in their lives.

6. ***Is your child using food as a weapon?***

A girl with a beautiful mother may overeat because that is the best way to avoid competition. A boy with a father who wants him to be an All-American may stuff himself with food so that he has an excuse for not going on the field and showing everyone that he really isn't good at sports.

Naturally, your child isn't going to *tell* you this. The child probably doesn't even understand why he does it. But you know your child better than anyone else does. If you watch his actions and think about his situation, you should be able to get a pretty good idea of whether or not your child is punishing you by getting fat.

7. ***Is your child driven by unconscious fears?***

Throughout the years at my camps, I have encountered the strange case of the child who swears that he wants to lose weight, but then does everything possible to keep himself from getting slimmer. I have come to the conclusion that to some children, subconsciously, being fat is a great advantage. The bigger body makes them seem stronger than they really are. They don't have to defend themselves in schoolyard fights. In addition, fat boys don't get chosen for teams; fat girls don't get invited to parties. Their parents may worry about them being left out, but for some fat children, outside is just where they want to be, thank you very much. If they're outside, they don't have to compete. They can amble along their merry way and no one will bother them.

If you suspect that your child uses his fatness as a defense against threatening situations, I suggest you seek professional help. Nothing you can do is going to be of use with the child who unconsciously is determined to remain fat.

At this point, I must warn you against trying to be your own psychiatrist. I've seen too many children desperately unhappy because their parents had been playing psychological tricks to get them to lose weight. Please, please, don't ever get into those threatening, bribing, pleading, cajoling routines that make life so miserable for the overweight child.

What I suggest is that you look at your child's eating habits and the habits of your family, and then try to understand why your child is overweight. If you come to the conclusion that there is a deep emotional reason why your child is overeating, then I urge you to seek competent, professional help for your child. It may be painful for everyone to begin with, but nothing else you can undertake will do any good if you ignore a child's deeply rooted emotional problems.

However, if you analyze the situation and decide that your child's weight problem is primarily the result of his bad eating habits and his environment, then *you* must teach your child good eating habits and change that environment.

2

Plain Talk

During precamp interviews, I have had many mothers tell me of their teen-age daughters' popularity. Then the girl arrives at camp, and I discover that she is feeling absolutely miserable.

Yes, all the pretty girls in the class want to have her for a friend. She's no competition for them. The pretty girl doesn't mind taking the overweight girl to parties or to informal gatherings where she wants to rely on safety in numbers. The pretty girl can only look better standing beside the fat girl.

Boys are often nice to the fat girl. She's sympathetic and pathetically eager for any attention they deign to bestow upon her. So they use her to help with the homework, to keep confidences, and frequently to carry messages to the pretty girls.

The fat girl often has several pals among the boys. But when it comes to romance, well, you can't expect a guy to actually take a fat girl out, can you? He might enjoy talking to her and he might even be attracted to her physically, but what would his friends say if he showed up with a fat girl in tow? At best, they'd think he was being charitable. At worst, they'd think he had something wrong with him. And no pretty girl would have anything to do with him. For children in early adolescence, nothing counts more than appearances. And I don't think there is anything in the world more cruel than the way young adolescents treat each other.

So don't be fooled if your overweight child is a pal to everybody. She—and in many cases he—is well aware of what is going on and how she is being used. And she hates it. But she puts up with it because when you are overweight and miserable, even friends you know to be false are better than no friends at all.

Often I am amazed at the amount of suffering loving parents can allow their children to endure. They want to help, they firmly believe they are helping, but they do not look at the world in the same way the child looks at it. They often don't see that parental help can do more harm than good.

I have drawn up a list of ten commandments for parents. If you keep these rules in mind, there is less chance that you will make your child's life miserable, and more chance that you will help him lose weight.

1. ***Thou Shalt Not Nag***

A child who wants to lose weight doesn't need to be reminded of his problem ten times a day. He'll control his eating habits to please himself. If he's not ready to begin a serious weight-control program, no amount of urging from his parents will help. The constant reminders of what he ought to do will just make it that much harder for him to do it when he's ready. He'll start to think of losing weight as showing weakness and "giving in." So don't let nagging turn weight control into a test of wills between you and your child.

2. ***Thou Shalt Not Be Sarcastic***

So often parents feel that if they deride their child often enough—especially in front of his friends and relatives—they'll inspire him to lose weight. They reason that their child will lose weight just to escape being made the butt of jokes. I have yet to meet a child who was helped by teasing and ridicule.

An overweight child doesn't need any encouragement to feel unhappy. He feels worthless enough without his parents and family reminding him that people don't like him because he's fat. When parents join the chorus of criticism, the child's worst fears are confirmed. He believes that because he is fat, there is nobody in the whole world he can trust. This feeling of rejection is so awful that it saps the child's strength, and he begins to retreat into his own world. Instead of strengthening his will to diet, sarcasm destroys it.

3. ***Thou Shalt Not Put A Price Tag On Your Love***

I've seen many parents give their child the message—sometimes directly but more often by the things they *don't* say—that they would love him more if only he weighed less. It's true that slender people seem more popular and enjoy a better social life—particularly in their teens. But parental love is something quite different from social popularity. At least it ought to be.

Your child needs your love and support all the time—especially when he's overweight and feels that the rest of the world doesn't understand him.

4. ***Thou Shalt Not Lock Up The Cookies And Candies***

Hiding sweet food challenges your child to find it. If you make sweet foods into a game, then naturally, your child will try to win it. And since you can't watch over him twenty-four hours a day, he probably *will* win it.

The only way to keep a child from eating fattening foods is to teach him self-control. And one of the best ways to begin is to place him on an honor system.

5. ***Thou Shalt Not Offer Bribes***

You offer your overweight little girl a new dress if she can reduce by a size or two. She says, "Yes, I am really going to try hard now." Somehow, she doesn't quite make it. She feels angry at herself because she failed. She may be so discouraged she gives up completely.

You're faced with a dilemma. If you give her the dress even though she didn't reach your objective, what was the point in setting one? If you refuse to give her the dress, then you're rejecting your daughter. It's better not to get caught in the trap of offering material rewards for losing weight.

6. ***Thou Shalt Take Your Child Into Your Confidence***

A child understands more than we think. When the family faces a financial crisis, when one member is handicapped physically, or when a father or mother is drinking so much that he or she is getting close to alcoholism, the youngster is well aware of the situation.

But if you don't admit the problem to the child, you force him to deal with it on his own. And if it's hard for you to cope with, imagine how much harder it must be for the child!

Is it any wonder, then, that the youngster turns to the solace of food and quickly eats himself into an overweight condition in such circumstances?

7. ***Thou Shalt Make Weight Control A Family Project***

When you focus a great deal of attention on one overweight child, you are certain to arouse some resentment from the other children in the family, particularly if they are younger. The child who is trying to lose weight feels this resentment, and it makes weight control that much harder. There is nothing more cruel than a sibling's teasing.

You should take your children into your confidence and ask for their cooperation. A little help and support from brothers and sisters can help make an overweight child feel he is loved and needed.

8. ***Thou Shalt Make Home Life As Stable As Possible***

All children dislike change, and adolescents dislike it most of all. The latter are just beginning a social life and suddenly father is transferred or the family prospers and buys a better house in another neighborhood. When this kind of natural "disaster" occurs in a child's life, it is the parents' responsibility to keep the child's routine as well balanced as possible. In some cases, it might even be advisable to let a child live with relatives or a good friend until a school term is completed, and then he can transfer to a new school with less disruption.

9. ***Thou Shalt Be A Paragon Of Patience***

Your child is bound to slip on a weight-control program. Inevitably, he's going to make mistakes about his diet and may even gain a little weight at some point. And he will probably feel worse than you. If you quietly ignore it, he'll probably resume the proper routine on his own.

10. ***Thou Shalt Be Wrong—At Least Some Of The Time***

No one is harder to live with than the person who is always right and always saying "I told you so!" If you admit to a child that you make mistakes, particularly with his weight-control program, then he won't feel so badly when he makes mistakes, too. He'll be more tolerant of you and of himself. After all, losing and controlling weight are living processes; they cannot be reduced to mechanical formulas. A child cannot lose weight according to rigid specifications. Once your child knows that you understand and accept this fact, then you've gone a long way toward making weight control a natural part of his life.

3

Motivation

My ten commandments for parents are a prescription for creating a warm, loving atmosphere for the child who is trying to lose weight. They are guidelines for creating the support that the child absolutely must have to take off and keep off pounds. But in themselves, the ten commandments won't help your child to lose weight. They are not motives.

Too often it is so obvious to the parents that the child must lose weight that they can't understand why the child doesn't put himself on a strict diet. But to the child, the reasons may not yet be apparent. The child hasn't been motivated. And until he really *wants* to lose weight, no diet can help him.

Until now, I've been discussing mostly what you must not do. This chapter is about what you can do to help your child *want* to lose weight.

1. ***Prove to him that he can lose weight***

Sometimes a change in routine can lead to a loss in weight. A child makes a team or lands a part in a play, and he puts so much time and energy into the project he forgets about food. Before he is aware of what is happening, he's managed to drop a few pounds.

I wouldn't make a big fuss on such occasions. But if you casually remark to your child that he looks a bit slimmer, he will get the point. He will realize that being fat is not a permanent condition. Without even trying, he lost weight. Imagine how much more he could lose if he really put his mind to it!

2. ***Don't be afraid to encourage romance***

Among my girl campers the most common reason given for wanting to lose weight is, of course, "a boy."

Among my boy campers, I think "a girl" is the most common reason for wanting to reduce. However, the boys are much more reluctant to admit it.

The problem for a mother is how to use that interest in the opposite sex without looking as though she's trying to push her daughter—or her son—into an early marriage. And social life is one area where children want absolutely no interference from adults.

I think the best thing a mother can do is to create a warm, pleasant atmosphere so that her children will feel completely at ease bringing their friends home. Rock music may drive you batty, but it can provide a good social setting for your children. With a son, encourage a sister to teach him the latest dance steps. Or if you must, learn them and then teach him yourself.

I'm not suggesting that you try to become a "pal" to your children. But if you can quietly nudge them into a more social world, their natural desire to play an active role can motivate them to lose weight.

3. ***Hang a few full-length mirrors around the house***

There's nothing like a good hard look at themselves to convince children that it's time to take off weight. The girl who tells herself she's just "pleasingly plump" and the boy who thinks that he's just a little "huskier" than his friends can get a rude shock when they are confronted by their mirror image.

4. ***Go for a little shopping trip***

The pleasingly plump girl who tries to buy a bathing suit will discover faster than words can convey that there's nothing pleasant about being overweight. The young man who pictures himself in a pair of dungarees and then discovers that the only pants that fit him would look better on his grandfather will be ready and eager to lose weight.

5. ***Find a talent and encourage it***

Most children have at least one thing they do well or one activity they would really like to try. The girl who is interested in modern dance and the boy who wants to take karate lessons are ripe for losing weight.

If you can get the youngster involved in a new activity that really absorbs his interest, you may find that you won't have to do anything else. Once he realizes that his participation will require special skills and good physical condition, he is ready to begin losing weight.

6. ***A chance to make a fresh start***

I mentioned earlier that moving from city to city or changing schools can prompt some children to withdraw from an active social life and cause them to gain weight. But a dramatic change can also provide them with a good opportunity to begin a new life, especially if it occurs during the summer before school starts. When other children have gotten used to thinking of someone as fat, it's sometimes hard for the child to imagine himself being thin. But if he's going to a new school where he knows no one, he has a fine chance to make a fresh start.

7. ***Get him involved in helping other people***

In every community there are many opportunities for public service, ranging from reading to older people or to the blind to working in a political campaign.

Too often, the heavy child indulges himself in self-pity. He's worthless, everybody knows he's worthless, and there's nobody in the whole world as badly off as he. Or so he tells himself. But when he gets involved in public service he often discovers that there are people who have far more

> serious troubles than he. And the feeling of self-pity becomes impossible to sustain.
>
> Realizing that he can help people in trouble, he finds new power within himself, power he may never have known existed. Instead of thinking of himself as the local slob, he has a new, confident self-image. And one of the first things he is likely to want to do is create the proper physical presence to go with the emotional picture he now has of himself.

I hope you notice one thing about all these suggestions to motivate your child to lose weight. They are all positive, they involve leading the child, not threatening, bribing, nagging or cajoling him. If you try to pressure your child into weight reduction, you'll build up a wall of resentment that may take years to break down.

There is a last category of motivation that I haven't included in the list because I don't really know how to define it. When I ask my campers why they decided to lose weight, many tell me they just can't remember. The feeling came over them one day and that was it. They had tried all kinds of diets and had some success, but then put all the weight back on. They had gone through the cycle of gorging themselves and claiming they were going on a diet "right after the holidays" or "as soon as school ends."

One day they made up their minds that they had to be serious about losing weight. And where they had been weak before, they were suddenly full of determination. The youngsters weren't very articulate about why they suddenly could do things that would have seemed an impossible exercise of willpower only a week or two before. But obviously, the climate for making such a decision must have been encouraging. And the home environment must have been very good.

One day, your child could make the decision to lose weight, too. That day will come a lot faster if you create the proper atmosphere.

4

Dieting Facts

It's important for you and your child to understand some of the things that are going to happen when he goes on a diet. Weight reducing is a physical process and it is going to produce some physical changes. You should also be on the lookout for a few emotional changes.

The first week can be discouraging as well as wildly encouraging. The child may lose weight spectacularly, but he may feel so bad that he'll wonder if it's really worth the trouble. During this time the body loses more water than at any other period of a diet. This decrease shows up on the scale, but it is a little misleading to think of it as a real weight loss. Still, pounds lost are lost pounds and your child will feel grateful about what is happening.

At the same time, he is likely to feel miserable. He's been used to eating what he wanted. Now he has to start saying no to himself. It will take some time for his appetite stimulators, the salivary glands, to get the message. They'll keep telling him he's hungry, and he'll have to keep telling himself he mustn't eat. The result can be the most appalling orgy of self-pity.

The best thing you can do is to keep promising your child that if he can get through the first week without yielding to temptation, the rest will be relatively easy. He's used to having his stomach feel full and even bloated; now it feels empty all the time. You have to convince him that if he leaves his stomach alone, it will make the adjustment without any help from him. After all, he knows that you are feeding him as many calories as he really needs. You're not trying to starve him.

He'll continue losing weight for several weeks and even months. But then, quite unexpectedly, he'll stop. He may go for weeks without losing another pound. And naturally enough, he'll start to feel discouraged and think that he's lost as much as he can. He may even want to give up the whole thing.

What is happening is that the body is getting used to its new fueling system. Once this is done, the dieting will be effective again.

It's impossible to predict just when the plateau will be reached. Or when the pounds will begin to disappear again. But be assured—and assure your child—that once he has crossed to the other side of the plateau, he will, indeed, continue to lose weight.

A teen-age girl can add as many as four or five pounds of excess water during the menstrual period. At this time, she is likely to be highly sensitive and moody, and the additional weight may make her want to give up the diet. However, if she knows what is happening to her body and she understands that the excess water will quickly disappear, she should get through these periods without too much disappointment.

If your child has been through the depressing cycle of losing weight and then gaining it back and more besides, he's going to wonder what's so different this time. I hope you will be able to make him understand why he has a better chance if he changes his whole style of life instead of just altering his eating habits. It might also help if you can explain why diets alone never really work. If he knows why he failed before, he will understand why he can succeed this time.

1. ***His earlier diets were unrealistic.***

   Fad or so-called "wonder" diets are based on the idea of

restricting a person to a limited group of foods for a certain period of time.

I can't emphasize too strongly my own personal dislike of fad diets. They are boring and they are futile. A person suffers with them for a period of time and may even lose some weight, but as soon as he gives up the "wonder" diet and goes back to "normal" living, he puts all the weight back on again—and then some.

In addition, fad diets may be injurious to the health of a growing child, particularly an adolescent. Children need a nutritionally balanced intake of food. If they don't get it, their physical development can be retarded and they can become ill.

2. ***Maybe dieting was too easy the first time.***

From time to time, I have met children who tell me they can take off weight any time they want. I've discovered that what has usually happened in these cases is that an overweight child goes on a diet and learns, much to his surprise, that losing weight was pretty easy. All that talk about diets being hard to stay on was so much nonsense spread about by adults who, everybody knows, aren't as strong minded and determined as children.

Once the child has proved to himself he can do it, he doesn't see any reason to continue. So he stops dieting, secure in the knowledge that he can start again whenever he so desires. In the meantime, there's no need to worry much about food. And the child begins gaining weight again —sometimes quite spectacularly.

It's vitally important to make your child understand that the object of dieting is not to prove he has good willpower. The name of the game is losing weight. And the only way to "win" this game is to keep off the weight.

3. ***Did he think he'd become a bean pole overnight?***

Some children, especially ones who have never gone on a diet before, think that all they have to do is control their intake of food for a couple of weeks and suddenly they will be models of slender grace. And, of course, when the formula doesn't work they get discouraged and they want to give up.

Make sure your child understands that beginning a diet is a long-term process. Don't let him think that he's going to lose ten pounds the first week and twenty-five pounds in the first month. As I said previously, two pounds a week is a reasonable weight-loss average to aim for.

Too often, children expect that if they can solve the problem of controlling their weight all their other problems will disappear, too. Unfortunately, real life is never that simple, especially for adolescents.

A young man must understand that losing weight will not make him a better athlete. It will give him the *potential* to become good at sports, but he will still have to work hard to develop his skills and make the football or basketball team.

And a young girl must understand that just because she's slimmer, the boys suddenly will not come flocking around her. The ability to talk easily, the ability to dance, the ability to discover and speak freely about a common interest with a boy, all these play their part in making a girl attractive to boys.

5

Calorie-Wise Shopping

Cooking is an art and in later chapters, you will find some recipes that can make diet eating a pleasure. But before we discuss cooking, I'd like to point out a few things about the raw materials and equipment you're going to need.

From now on, supermarket shopping will be a different experience. At the end of this chapter, you'll find a very good calorie guide—take it with you when you go shopping. You have to learn to calculate calories as carefully as you watch prices.

For instance, you'll sometimes see a box of wafers marked "Only 4 calories per serving." This means that there are only four calories in one perforated, bite-sized square. The wafer is mostly air and your child could easily go through a whole box in one sitting and still feel hungry.

Watch out for foods labeled "for dietetic use." This phrase can mean low in calories or it can mean salt-free or sugar-free for diabetic use. The latter can still be loaded with fat-producing carbohydrates. Check the label for mention of "manitol," "hexitol" or "sorbitol." These are sugar substitutes that have as many carbohydrates as sugar. Also keep in mind that any ingredient ending in "ose" such as dextrose, maltose, or sucrose is a form of sugar.

Until the cyclamate scare a few years ago, artificially sweetened foods were a fad as big as health foods are now. The possibility that cyclamates in extra-large doses might cause cancer has made many people think twice before using any artificial sweeteners.

It's hard to live without the taste of something sweet during the day. But the trick is to educate your child to accept the natural sweetness that he can find in fruit as a substitute for sugar or artificial sweeteners.

At my camps we only use artificial sweetener in the morning cocoa, when the children want a hot drink that will wake them up. The remainder of the day we rely on natural foods. At snack times, we give them apples or carrots or bananas. If they're thirsty and want something a little tastier than a glass of water, we give them an orange.

Some people try to discourage dieters from drinking water because they believe the body retains it; but this isn't true. We encourage children to drink as much water as they want. Water is necessary for good digestion and it really doesn't matter how much dieting children drink. The only time I try to restrain them is before and after meals. If they drink too much at either time, they will wash the food through their systems before the body has had a chance to absorb the nourishment.

I don't rely on canned or frozen fruit juices. Too often, they have been dosed with sugar or artificial sweeteners. I would rather teach children to quench their thirst with fresh fruit juice. It's richer in vitamins, it tastes better, and it provides enough bulk in their stomachs to still any hunger pangs that may occur between meals.

After years of experimenting with different, artificially sweetened, and supposedly low-calorie canned fruits, I've found a simple way to save myself the trouble. For some reason the low-calorie canned fruits do not taste as good as the regular canned fruits. Now I buy the latter and pour off the calorie-rich syrup. Fortunately, very little of the syrup's sugar has penetrated the fruit. I pour ice water over the fruit so that it can be served in a liquid.

When you are buying meat, stay away from all those lovely marbled cuts. The marble is fat and it's supposed to help the meat cook and taste better. I find both these ideas dubious. There is no taste in fat, and low-calorie oil can help your meat cook just as well.

Veal, then lean beef, ground, or otherwise, are your best values in low-calorie meats. Chickens and turkeys are both good and inexpensive.

Please don't buy packaged hamburger. I know it's often sold at bargain prices, but if it puts more weight on your child, it's no bargain at all.

Stay away from lunch meats or fish canned in oil such as sardines. Also cross off meat sauces, pork and beans, chilis, and canned stews. These "convenience" foods can make life very inconvenient for you in the future when they add pounds to your child. All canned meats and meat sauces are packed with fat.

Dry cereals in the morning are a habit with many families, and I don't try to change that practice at my camps. But I do try to give the children the new dry cereals that are advertised as high in protein and low in calories. And I always serve the cereals with skim milk and a little artificial sweetener so the children who feel the need for something sweet will have it on the breakfast table. Cereals are very fattening when they are combined with whole milk and sugar. There are no more than fifty calories in a cup of puffed rice or puffed wheat, but when either is combined with milk and sugar, the calorie content zooms.

Many people feel that cheese is a good source of protein and therefore, if they eat a lot of cheese instead of meat, they are cutting down on their intake of calories. Unfortunately, this isn't necessarily so.

Pot cheese, for instance, is a great favorite of dieters but it is rich in calories, and, of course, so is cream cheese. If you like this style of cheese, look for farmer cheese at your supermarket. It tastes the same as cream cheese but it has half the calories.

The cheese lowest in calories is still that faithful friend of the dieter—cottage cheese. At my camps, I rely on it heavily. It tastes good, and when it comes to something rich in food value and low in calories, nothing beats this cheese.

Many people are still reluctant to use powdered milk. They

think of it as a poor man's food and they tell themselves that even if they do have to budget carefully, they can afford to drink whole milk. Actually, they are missing out on one of the most valuable foods for dieters. Powdered milk is lowest in calories, and when mixed and thoroughly chilled, I think it tastes better than skim milk or any milk substitute presently on the market.

Snacks are the perennial and inescapable problem for the parent of a dieting child. At my camps I have a snack shop, and the campers may buy 50¢ worth of sugarless gum or candy every week. I've learned through hard experience that the habit of reaching for a snack is so deeply ingrained in our children that it's futile to attempt to cure them of it completely.

However, I try to get the youngsters to accept fruit as a substitute for candy. And when the craving for candy or gum overcomes them, I make sure that all the sweet things the campers purchase at the candy store are as sugarless as the manufacturers can make them. There is a whole range of sugarless confections ranging from soda pop to chewing gum, and I suggest you keep a few of these on hand. It's better, of course, to seduce them with some vegetables or fruit but it's also a good idea to know when to give in. It's a wise parent who knows her own child.

A final word about cooking: You're going to need some specialized kitchen equipment. Here are some items I have found useful when cooking for a child trying to lose weight.

A heavy teflon skillet: This utensil can save you a whopping 100 calories for every teaspoonful of oil you would normally use for frying. And the food looks—and tastes—as though it had been broiled.

A blender: This can be an expensive initial investment, but it will soon pay for itself with all the low-calorie dressings, sauces, and drinks you can prepare.

A meat grinder: Prepared meats and sandwich fillers have extremely fattening ingredients. Even the dietetic sandwich fillers contain "stretchers" that are heavy with carbohydrates. With a meat grinder, you can use leftovers to make your own sandwich fillings and keep your child's calorie intake down—as well as stretching your own budget.

An electric slicer: The thinner you slice meat, bread, and other foods the better. Three thin slices of beef may look like more than one thick slice that weighs, in fact, three times as much.

A bacon crisper: Bacon, obviously, is not a food I would recommend to a child on a diet. But I have found children who are positively addicted to their morning bacon. If your child is a "bacon head," cook the bacon in a crisper. It drains off the fat and keeps the bacon from curling. And it's not as fattening as bacon fried in a pan.

An egg poacher: This will enable you to cook eggs without butter, another savings in calories.

Glass baking dishes: You can undertake nonfat cooking with these better than with metal cooking trays.

A vegetable shredder: The hand will do quite nicely for chopping up vegetables. But if you have a large family, an electric shredder with quick-changing blades can save you a lot of time.

Molds: Ring and fruit molds are basic, but it helps if you have a variety of shapes and sizes. They will enable you to make many low-calorie dishes with gelatins and aspics.

A pastry tube: A few squiggles of low-calorie topping can make the most ordinary dessert seem like an expedition into delicious self-indulgence.

CALORIE CHART

Food	Serving Size	Approximate Calories
Apple	1 large	100
Apple, baked (with sugar)	1 large	200
Apple butter	1 tablespoon	40
Apple juice (cider)	1 cup (8 ounces)	125
Applesauce:		
sweetened	1 cup	184
unsweetened	1 cup	100
Apricots:		
canned (with heavy syrup)	4 medium halves	100
dried	4 large halves	60
raw	3 medium	52
Artichoke	1 medium	75
Asparagus, canned or fresh	8 medium spears	26
Avocado	½ medium pear	200
with salad dressing		380
Bacon	2 slices	100
Bagel	1 medium	180
Bamboo shoots	1 cup	40
Banana	1 small	60
Beans:		
baked, canned, pork-tomato sauce	1 cup	350
snap, fresh or canned	1 cup	50
kidney, canned	1 cup	200
lima, fresh or canned	1 cup	160
Bean sprouts, cooked	1 cup	63
Beef, cooked:		
chuck, without bone	3 ounces	250
corned	3 ounces, 1 slice	150
dried	2 ounces	110
hamburger patty	3 ounces	275
hamburger patty (lean)	3 ounces	200
porterhouse	3 ounces	275
roast (lean)	3 ounces	175
sirloin (lean)	3 ounces	250
stew	1 cup	400

Food	Serving Size	Approximate Calories
Beet greens	1 cup	50
Beets	1 cup	75
Biscuits:		
baking powder	1 (2-inch diameter)	85
refrigerator	1 biscuit	70
Blackberries	1 cup	90
Blueberries, fresh or frozen, no sugar	1 cup	90
Bluefish, baked	4 ounces	175
Bologna	1 slice	100
Bouillon cubes	1 cube	6
Bread:		
brown	1 slice	100
corn	1 piece	160
cracked wheat	1 slice	80
Melba toast	1 slice	20
rye	1 slice	65
white	1 slice	65
whole-wheat	1 slice	75
Bread crumbs:		
dry, packaged	1 cup	300
fresh	1 cup	90
Broccoli	1 cup	20
Brownies	1 2-inch square by 1 inch	190
Brussels sprouts	6 sprouts	60
Buns:		
cinnamon	1 large	350
hot cross	1 medium	185
Butter	1 tablespoon	100
Buttermilk	1 cup (8 ounces)	85
Cabbage:		
cooked	½ cup	20
raw	½ cup shredded	10
Cakes:		
angel food	1 2-inch wedge	110
cheesecake (cream cheese base)	1 slice, ⅛ of cake	450
chiffon	10-inch cake, 1/16 of cake	295

Food	Serving Size	Approximate Calories
chocolate layer cake, fudge frosting	2 layers, 1/12 of cake	435
cupcake, 7-minute frosting	1 medium	205
fruit cake	9-inch round cake, 1/32 of cake	310
pound cake	1 slice 3 x 5½ inches	210
sponge cake	9-inch tube cake, 1/12 of cake	125
white layer cake, butter frosting	2 9-inch layers, 1/16 of cake	325
Candy:		
bar, average	1 average	295
caramel, plain	1 small piece	40
chocolate cream	1 medium piece	50
chocolate, milk	1 ounce	145
chocolate mint	1 patty, 1-inch diameter	35
fondant	1 ounce	100
fudge (with nuts)	1 piece, 1-inch square	75
gumdrops	1 small	10
hard candy	1 large sour ball	35
Life-savers	1 saver	10
peanut brittle	1 ounce	125
Cantaloupe	½	35
Carrots:		
cooked	½ cup, diced	20
raw	1 small	25
Catsup, chili sauce	1 tablespoon	15
Cauliflower, cooked	1 cup	30
Celery	1 large stalk	10
Cereals, cooked:		
corn meal, yellow or white	¾ cup, cooked	90
farina or granular wheat	¾ cup, cooked	100
rolled oats	¾ cup, cooked	100
Cereals, ready-to-eat:		
corn, rice, wheat flakes	1 cup (about 1 ounce)	95
puffed (rice, wheat)	1 cup (about ½ ounce)	50
shredded wheat	1 large biscuit or ½ cup bite sized	150

Food	Serving Size	Approximate Calories
wheat bran (100%)	1 cup	145
Cheese:		
American cheddar (processed or natural)	1 slice (1 ounce)	105
Camembert	1 ounce	85
cottage, creamed	1 cup	230
plain	1 cup	200
cream	*see* Milk	
mozzarella	1 ounce	110
Parmesan or Romano, grated	2 tablespoons (¼ ounce)	55
ricotta, partially skim milk	⅓ cup	85
whole milk	⅓ cup	120
Roquefort or blue	1 ounce	105
spread, processed	1 ounce	80
Swiss (processed or natural)	1 slice (1 ounce)	105
Cheese soufflé	1 serving, about 1½ cups	320
Cherries:		
canned in syrup	½ cup, 3 tablespoons syrup	110
canned, red sour, pitted	1 cup	120
fresh, sweet	1 cup	90
Chewing gum	1 stick	10
Chicken:		
croquette	1 medium	220
fryer, breast	1 whole small (¾ pound)	300
fryer, leg and thigh	1 small (½ pound)	190
roasted, no bone	average serving (4 ounces)	225
à la king	1 cup, no biscuit	375
pie (with biscuit topping)	¼ of a pie	585
Chili con carne	1 cup	320
Chocolate:		
semisweet	1 ounce	145
sweetened	1 ounce	150
unsweetened	1 ounce	145
Chocolate milk drink	1 glass (8 ounces)	240
Chocolate syrup	1 tablespoon	40

Food	Serving Size	Approximate Calories
Chop suey over rice	1 cup suey, ½ cup rice	535
Cider, sweet	1 cup (8 ounces)	125
Clams, raw	6 (4 ounces, meat only)	90
Cocoa, prepared with milk	1 cup	235
Coconut:		
dried, shredded, sweetened	½ cup	175
fresh, shredded	½ cup	175
Coffee, without sugar and cream	1 cup	0
Coffee cake (with nuts)	1 piece, 2 x 3½ inches	250
Cola drinks	6 ounces	75
Collards, cooked	½ cup	40
Cookies:		
chocolate chip	1 ½-inch diameter	70
fig bar	1 ½-inch square bar	55
macaroon	1 2½-inch diameter	70
oatmeal	1 3-inch diameter	80
sugar	1 3-inch diameter	80
sugar wafer	1 2½ x ¾-inch rectangle	25
Corn:		
canned, whole kernel	½ cup	70
fresh	1 ear, 5 inches long, 1¾-inch diameter	85
Corn fritters	1 small, 2-inch diameter	45
Corn meal, dry	1 cup	525
Cornstarch	1 tablespoon	30
Crabmeat, fresh, frozen, or canned	½ cup (2¼ ounces)	75
Crackers:		
graham	4 small	56
oyster	1 cup	120
round	1 cracker	15
saltine	1 2-inch square	15
soda	1 2½-inch square	25
whole rye	1 double cracker	20
Cranberries, raw	1 cup	55
Cranberry juice	½ cup	75
Cranberry sauce, sweetened, canned	1 tablespoon	35

Food	Serving Size	Approximate Calories
Cream:		
half and half	1 tablespoon	20
heavy	1 tablespoon	50
light	1 tablespoon	30
sour, commercial	1 tablespoon	30
Creamed fish	1 cup serving	415
Cucumbers, uncooked	6 slices, ⅛-inch thick	5
Currants, raw	½ cup	30
Custard, baked or boiled	½ cup	140
Custard, frozen	½ cup	200
Dandelion greens, cooked	½ cup	40
Danish pastry	1 medium	225
Dates, dried	¼ cup	125
Dessert topping (brands vary)	1 tablespoon	10 to 25
Doughnuts:		
cake-type	1 medium	135
jelly	1 medium	185
Duck, cooked	½ small	375
Eclair, iced (custard filling)	1 medium	565
Eggnog	1 glass (8 ounces)	250
Eggplant, uncooked	1 slice, 5 inches diameter	20
Eggs:		
fried	1 egg, 1 teaspoon fat or oil	105
omelet	2 eggs, 2 teaspoons butter	215
raw	1 medium	75
white	1 medium	15
yolk	1 medium	60
scrambled	2 eggs, 2 tablespoons milk, 2 tablespoons butter	275
shirred or poached	1 medium	75
Endive, raw	2 stalks	25
Escarole, raw	4 leaves	20
Figs, dried	1 large	55
Finnan haddie	4 ounces	120
Flounder, raw	4 ounces	80

Food	Serving Size	Approximate Calories
Flour:		
all-purpose	1 cup, sifted	400
cake	1 cup, sifted	365
whole-wheat	1 cup, sifted	400
Frankfurter	1 medium	125
French toast	1 slice, no syrup	140
Fruit cocktail, canned	½ cup fruit and syrup	90
Garlic	1 clove	3
Gelatin dessert	½ cup	75
Gelatins, unflavored	1 envelope	30
Ginger ale	1 glass (8 ounces)	80
Gingerbread	3 inches square (unfrosted)	345
Goose, cooked	4 ounces	265
Grapefruit	½ medium	75
Grapefruit juice:		
sweetened, canned	½ cup	65
unsweetened, fresh, frozen, or canned	½ cup	45
Grapefruit sections	½ cup, 1 tablespoon syrup	90
Grape juice	½ cup	85
Grapes	20 medium	50
Gravy:		
cream	2 tablespoons	45
regular (from broth)	2 tablespoons	25
Griddle cakes	1 4-inch diameter (no syrup)	100
Haddock, pan-fried	1 fillet (3½ ounces)	160
Halibut, broiled	1 steak (4½ ounces)	230
Hash, corned-beef, canned	1 cup (3 ounces)	120
Herring, smoked	3 ounces	180
Honey	1 tablespoon	60
Honeydew melon	2-inch wedge from 6½ by 7-inch melon	50
Ice cream (vanilla)	½ cup or ⅛ of quart	200
Ice cream soda, vanilla	1 regular	270
Ice milk	½ cup or ⅛ of quart	135
Jam	1 tablespoon	55

Food	Serving Size	Approximate Calories
Jelly	1 tablespoon	50
Junket	½ cup	125
Kale, cooked	½ cup	25
Lamb, cooked:		
chop, with bone	4 ounces	315
roast, no bone	3 ounces	230
Lard	1 tablespoon	125
Lasagna	4½ x 2½-inch serving	785
Lemon juice, fresh, frozen, or canned	1 ounce	8
Lemonade concentrate, frozen	1 cup (8 ounces)	100
Lentils, dried, uncooked	½ cup	200
Lettuce, raw	3 large leaves	10
Liver:		
beef, cooked	2 ounces	120
calf, raw	3 ounces	120
chicken, raw	3 ounces	120
Liverwurst	2 ounces	150
Lobster, canned or fresh	½ cup (3 ounces)	80
Loganberries	½ cup	45
Luncheon meat, canned	1 slice (1 ounce)	80
Macaroni, cooked	½ cup	105
Macaroni and cheese	1 serving, about 1 cup	560
Margarine	1 tablespoon	100
Margarine, diet	1 tablespoon	50
Marmalade	1 tablespoon	55
Marshmallow, plain	1 average	25
Matzo:		
egg	1 regular	125
plain	1 regular	100
Meat loaf	1 serving 5 x 3 x 1-inch piece	335
Milk:		
buttermilk	1 glass (8 ounces)	85
condensed, sweetened	½ cup	490
evaporated	½ cup (undiluted)	175
half and half	½ cup	165
liquid, skim	1 glass (8 ounces)	85
whole	1 glass (8 ounces)	165

Food	Serving Size	Approximate Calories
malted (dry powder)	3 tablespoons (1 ounce)	125
nonfat dry milk, instant	½ cup	60
Milk shake	1 glass (8 ounces)	425
Molasses, light	1 tablespoon	50
Muffins:		
blueberry	1 2½-inch diameter	140
bran	1 2½-inch diameter	100
corn	1 2½-inch diameter	145
English	1 3½-inch diameter	130
plain	1 2½-inch diameter	115
Mushrooms:		
canned	1 cup (solids and liquids)	30
fresh	4 large	10
Noodles, cooked	½ cup	55
Noodles, chow mein, crisp, canned	1 cup	215
Oils, corn, cottonseed, olive, peanut, soybean	1 tablespoon	125
Okra, cooked	8 pods	30
Olives:		
green, unstoned	3 medium	20
ripe, unstoned	3 medium	30
Onion, raw	1 medium	52
Orange	1 medium, 3-inch diameter	70
Orange juice, fresh, frozen, canned	½ cup	55
Orange sections	½ cup	45
Parsley, raw	5 tablespoons, snipped	5
Parsnips, cooked	½ cup	45
Peaches, canned, syrup pack	2 halves, 2 tablespoons syrup	80
fresh	1 medium	45
frozen, sweetened	½ cup	90
Peach nectar	½ cup	55
Peanut butter	1 tablespoon	90
Peanuts	8 to 10	50
Pear nectar	½ cup	60

Food	Serving Size	Approximate Calories
Pears:		
canned, syrup pack	2 halves, 2 tablespoons syrup	80
fresh	1 medium	90
Peas:		
green, canned	½ cup	70
fresh, cooked	½ cup	55
split, dried and cooked	½ cup	345
Pecans	9 medium nuts	95
Peppers, green, raw	1 medium	15
Pickles:		
dill	1 large	15
sour	1 large	15
sweet	1 medium	20
Piecrust:		
double crust	1 9-inch diameter	2440
single crust	1 9-inch diameter	1220
Pies:		
apple (double crust)	3½-inch wedge (⅛ of 9-inch pie)	475
blueberry (double crust)	3½-inch wedge (⅛ of 9-inch pie)	440
cherry (double crust)	3½-inch wedge (⅛ of 9-inch pie)	475
coconut custard	3½-inch wedge (⅛ of 9-inch pie)	300
lemon meringue	3½-inch wedge (⅛ of 9-inch pie)	340
pecan	3½-inch wedge (⅛ of 9-inch pie)	570
pumpkin	3½-inch wedge (⅛ of 9-inch pie)	355
Pineapple:		
crushed, canned	½ cup	100
fresh, sliced	1 ¾-inch slice	45
juice, unsweetened	½ cup	60
sliced, canned	1 slice, ¾ inch thick 2 tablespoons syrup	95

Food	Serving Size	Approximate Calories
Pizza (with meat sauce and cheese)	¼ of 12-inch pie	575
Plums	1 2-inch diameter	30
Popcorn, unbuttered	1 cup	55
Popover	1 medium	120
Pork:		
ham, fresh, uncooked, no bone (with separable fat removed)	3 ounces	130
loin chop, uncooked, fat removed	4 ounces	215
Potatoes:		
baked or boiled	1 medium	95
chips	5 medium	50
French fried	8 pieces, 2x½x½ inches	155
hash browned	½ cup	235
scalloped	½ cup	120
sweet, baked or boiled	1 medium	185
sweet, candied	1 small, 3½x2¼ inches	315
white, mashed	½ cup (3 tablespoons milk, 1 tablespoon butter)	120
Poultry stuffing	1 cup	195
Pretzels	1 small, 1x2 inches or 5 2-inch sticks	20
Prune juice, canned	½ cup	85
Prunes:		
stewed and sweetened	4 with 2 tablespoons syrup	120
uncooked	4 medium	75
Puddings, made with whole milk:		
chocolate	½ cup	175
vanilla and butterscotch	½ cup	170
Pumpkin	½ cup	40
Pumpkin seeds:		
shelled	1 tablespoon	60
unshelled	¼ cup	40

Food	Serving Size	Approximate Calories
Radishes, raw	4 small	5
Raisins, seedless	¼ cup	110
Raspberries:		
black, fresh	½ cup	50
red, fresh	½ cup	35
Rhubarb:		
stewed and sweetened	½ cup	190
uncooked	1 cup	20
Rice:		
brown, uncooked	½ cup raw (about 1½ cups cooked)	375
precooked, dry	½ cup (makes 1 cup cooked)	200
white, uncooked	½ cup	345
cooked	½ cup	100
wild, uncooked	½ cup	295
Rice Krispies	1 cup	105
Rice pudding	¾ cup	225
Rolls, plain	1 small	80
	1 medium	125
	1 large	180
Rye wafers	1 wafer	22
Salads:		
apple, carrot with mayonnaise	½ cup	100
avocado-tomato-cottage cheese with French dressing	¼ avocado, ½ tomato, 2 tablespoons cheese, and 2 tablespoons dressing	305
cole slaw	½ cup	80
chicken, celery, mayonnaise	½ cup (1 tablespoon mayonnaise)	235
crab and celery with mayonnaise	½ cup (1 tablespoon mayonnaise)	185
cream cheese-pineapple with French dressing	1 slice pineapple,	

Food	Serving Size	Approximate Calories
	2 tablespoons cream cheese, 1 tablespoon dressing	215
lettuce	2 large leaves	7
mixed fruit (orange and grapefruit sections, grapes, canned peach, pineapple, 1 tablespoon orange juice, no dressing)	½ cup	70
mixed greens with French dressing	1 cup (1 tablespoon French dressing)	75
orange-grapefruit, French dressing	4 slices orange, 3 sections grapefruit, 1 tablespoon dressing	140
potato with mayonnaise	½ cup (1 tablespoon mayonnaise)	130
salmon and celery with mayonnaise	½ cup (1 tablespoon mayonnaise)	235
shrimp and celery with mayonnaise	1 cup (1 tablespoon mayonnaise)	250
tomato and lettuce (without dressing)		40
Waldorf and mayonnaise	½ cup (1 tablespoon mayonnaise)	125
Salad dressings:		
blue or Roquefort	1 tablespoon	75
French	1 tablespoon	60
Italian	1 tablespoon	85
mayonnaise	1 tablespoon	90
Russian	1 tablespoon	75
cooked type	1 tablespoon	75
Thousand Island	1 tablespoon	75
Salmon:		
baked	1 steak (4 ounces)	205
canned (sockeye or red)	½ cup, flaked (3 ounces)	145

Food	Serving Size	Approximate Calories
Sandwiches (calories are calculated on basis that bread is white or toast):		
bacon, lettuce, tomato	2 strips bacon, lettuce, tomato, 1 tablespoon mayonnaise	345
cheese (American, cheddar, Swiss)	1 slice cheese, 1 tablespoon mayonnaise	335
chicken salad	with lettuce ¼ cup filling	300
cream cheese and jelly	with 1½ tablespoons cheese, ½ tablespoon jelly	240
egg salad	1 egg, lettuce, 2 tablespoons mayonnaise	270
frankfurter on roll	1 frankfurter	245
ham, boiled	1 slice ham, lettuce, 1 tablespoon mayonnaise	310
ham and cheese	1 slice ham, 1 slice cheese, 1 tablespoon mayonnaise	420
hamburger on roll	3 ounces hamburger	440
lettuce and tomato	3 slices tomato, lettuce, 1½ teaspoons mayonnaise	190
peanut butter	1½ tablespoons peanut butter	270
peanut butter, jelly	1½ tablespoons peanut butter, 1½ teaspoons jelly	290
Sardines, canned in oil	4 medium	75
Sauces:		
barbecue	¼ cup	90
butterscotch	2 tablespoons	85
chocolate	2 tablespoons	105
hard	2 tablespoons	100
hollandaise	2 tablespoons	185
meat	¾ cup	325
tomato puree, canned	½ cup	45
white, medium	½ cup	210

Food	Serving Size	Approximate Calories
Sauerkraut	1 cup	32
Sausage, cooked, link	1 3½-inch long	75
Scallops, uncooked	4 ounces	88
Sherbet	½ cup	210
Shortening, hydrogenated	1 tablespoon	110
Shrimps, shelled, uncooked	4 ounces	140
Soft drinks (carbonated)	8 ounces	100
Soups:		
asparagus, cream of, canned (with milk)	¾ cup	120
bean, black, canned	¾ cup	80
beef noodle, canned	¾ cup	60
bouillon, canned	¾ cup	10
bouillon cube (chicken, beef, vegetable)	¾ cup	3 to 6
chicken, cream of, canned (with milk)	¾ cup	145
chicken gumbo, canned	¾ cup	45
chicken with rice, canned	¾ cup	35
clam chowder, Manhattan, canned	¾ cup	65
consommé, canned	1 cup	30
minestrone, canned	¾ cup	85
mushroom, cream of, canned	¾ cup	115
onion, canned	¾ cup	50
pea, green, canned	¾ cup	115
tomato, canned:		
clear	¾ cup	70
cream of	¾ cup	140
turkey noodle, canned	¾ cup	65
vegetable, canned	¾ cup	65
vichyssoise	1 cup	370
Spaghetti, cooked	¾ cup	100
Spinach, fresh, cooked	1 cup	46
Squash:		
summer, cooked	½ cup	15
winter, cooked	½ cup	45
Starch (arrowroot, corn, etc.)	1 tablespoon	30

Food	Serving Size	Approximate Calories
Strawberries:		
fresh	½ cup	25
frozen, sweetened	½ cup	120
Strawberry shortcake	1 serving with whipped cream	465
Stuffed pepper with meat, creole sauce	1 pepper	395
Succotash	½ cup	75
Sugar:		
brown	1 tablespoon	50
granulated	1 teaspoon	17
powdered (confectioners')	1 tablespoon	30
Sundaes:		
chocolate ice cream with chocolate sauce and chipped pecans	½ cup ice cream, 2 tablespoons sauce, and 2 tablespoons chopped pecans	405
vanilla ice cream with butterscotch sauce	½ cup ice cream, 2 tablespoons sauce	285
Sunflower seeds:		
shelled	1 tablespoon	45
unshelled	¼ cup	45
Sweetbreads, calves, raw	½ cup	115
Sweet potatoes	*see* Potatoes	
Swordfish, cooked	1 steak (4 ounces)	225
Syrup:		
maple	1 tablespoon	50
table (corn)	1 tablespoon	55
Tangerine	1 2½-inch diameter	35
Tangerine juice, unsweetened	1 cup	95
Tapioca (quick-cooking)	¼ cup	25
Tea, without sugar or cream	1 cup	0
Tomato juice	½ cup (4 ounces)	25

Food	Serving Size	Approximate Calories
Tomatoes:		
canned	½ cup	25
fresh	1 medium	30
Tongue, cooked	3 medium slices	100
Trout, rainbow, uncooked	4 ounces	225
Tuna:		
canned in oil	⅔ cup, drained	170
canned in water or broth-pack	¾ cup (3 ounces)	110
Turkey, raw	4 ounces	280
Turnips, white, cooked	½ cup	20
Veal:		
cutlet, uncooked	3 ounces	185
roast, cooked	1 slice (3 ounces)	195
Vegetable juice, canned	½ cup (4 ounces)	30
Vienna sausage, canned	4 ounces	245
Waffle	1 4½-inch square	120
Walnuts, chopped	1 tablespoon	50
Watercress, raw	1 small bunch	25
Watermelon	1 slice, 12 x 1 inch thick	70
Wheat flakes	1 cup	125
Wheat germ	1 tablespoon	15
Wheat, shredded	1 large biscuit	50
Yogurt	1 cup	130

6

Calorie-Counter Menus

The essential ingredients of diet cooking are imagination and efficiency. Using the calorie counter, you can let your imagination run free to prepare tasty and attractive meals. But you must be very efficient about calculating the amount of calories per ounce, teaspoon, tablespoon, and cupful. Portion control is vital to a diet. The average serving of meat is from three to four ounces. The average serving of a vegetable is one-half cup. When you increase these amounts, you are increasing the number of calories in your child's diet.

In this chapter, you will find a series of properly balanced and calorie-counted menus ranging from 900 to 2,000 calories a day. These consist of basic dishes which are easy to prepare as well as those which will require your imagination.

When you take your child for a pre-diet physical, your doctor may recommend a specific calorie intake for him. But I have found that 1,500 calories a day is a safe minimum requirement for a growing child. A variety of menus will allow you to average his calorie intake over a week, giving you some day-to-day leeway.

For example, if your child is going to a party or an outing with his friends, he will probably find it impossible to watch his diet. You can restrict him to 900 calories a day for the next few days in order to reach the desired balance for the week.

These diets permit flexibility, which is often a magic word when dealing with children.

900—Calorie Menus

No. 1

Breakfast	¼ cup fresh or canned diet raspberries 1 ounce or ½ thin slice broiled ham ½ toasted roll with 1 teaspoon diet jam 1 glass powdered milk
Lunch	Chicken liver sautéed with consommé Cauliflower with lemon, tomato, and lettuce salad, venegar and oil or diet dressing 3 diet plums in juice 1 glass skim milk
Dinner	4-ounce slice baked fresh salmon Stewed celery with diet butter seasoning Fresh asparagus Tossed green salad with diet dressing Sliced orange

No. 2

Breakfast	½ sliced banana 2 small Shredded Wheat biscuits 1 glass skim milk
Lunch	Beef stew (2 ounces beef) with small onion, carrot, and celery Pickled beet salad dotted with egg yellows ½ cup sherbet
Dinner	Clear chicken consommé Fresh fruit platter: sliced fresh pineapple, ½ cup fresh strawberries, ½ sliced orange, and ½ sliced peach 4 tablespoons cottage cheese and 1 double Ry-Krisp 1 glass powdered milk

No. 3

Breakfast	Large glass vegetable or tomato juice ½ cup Ralston 1 glass skim milk
Lunch	Bouillon Shrimp salad: 6 shrimps, ¼ cup celery, 2 egg whites, and diet dressing Carrot sticks Royal Ann or diet cherries 1 glass powdered milk or buttermilk
Dinner	3-ounce broiled beef patty Shredded zucchini Whole baby beets Tossed green salad with diet dressing ½ cup sliced fresh pineapple 1 glass skim milk

No. 4

Breakfast	Small glass unsweetened pineapple juice Baked French toast with 1 slice bread, 2 egg whites 1 glass powdered milk
Lunch	Clear chicken consommé 2 ounces or ¼ can diet tuna on bed of lettuce with carrot sticks, dill pickle, and quartered tomato with diet dressing Small baked apple 1 low-calorie soft drink
Dinner	Broiled lamb chop, fat trimmed ½ cup broccoli ½ cup carrots Cole slaw with diet dressing 3 small or 2 large fresh apricots 1 glass skim milk

No. 5

Breakfast
½ grapefruit
1 cup cereal
¼ slice dry toast
1 glass skim milk

Lunch
Clear consommé
Broiled filet of sole
½ cup broccoli
1 glass powdered milk or buttermilk
¾ cup artificially sweetened strawberries

Dinner
1 cup mixed vegetable juice
2 slices (¼ inch thick) canned corn beef
1 cup steamed cabbage
½ cup diced fresh pineapple with mint

No. 6

Breakfast
Small glass orange juice
½ slice whole wheat toast
2 tablespoons cottage cheese
1 glass powdered milk

Lunch
Tomato juice cocktail with 2 Ry-Krisps
Corned beef hash
String beans
Pickled beet salad
2 halves diet pears
1 glass powdered milk

Dinner
½ baked breast of chicken
Baked banana squash
Fresh spinach with lemon
Tomato salad with diet dressing
Low-calorie dessert with ½ sliced banana
1 glass powdered milk

No. 7

Breakfast	½ grapefruit, artificially sweetened Soft-boiled egg 1 Ry-Krisp and diet jam 1 glass powdered milk
Lunch	1 cup bouillon Vegetable plate with cooked cauliflower, green beans, and asparagus Cottage cheese and pimientos Flavored low-calorie gelatin 1 low-calorie soft drink
Dinner	1 small broiled chicken breast 1 broiled tomato 1 small (or ½) baked potato with salt Wedge of lettuce with low-calorie mayonnaise 3 canned low-calorie peaches Melba toast 1 glass powdered milk

No. 8

Breakfast	Half cantaloupe Scrambled egg ½ piece toast with diet margarine 1 glass powdered milk
Lunch	4 ounces drained tuna mixed with lettuce, celery, scallions, and string beans Low-calorie French dressing Ry-Krisp and small piece farmer cheese 1 diet cola
Dinner	Meatballs ½ cup cooked noodles 1 serving broccoli 1 cup bite-sized chicory with low-calorie dressing 2 diet-pack pear halves 1 glass powdered milk

No. 9

Breakfast	Sections of half an orange Dry cereal, artificially sweetened 1 glass powdered milk
Lunch	Chicken noodle soup Egg salad with diet mayonnaise 1 piece toast Flavored low-calorie gelatin 1 diet soft drink
Dinner	1 4-ounce broiled loin lamb chop 1 cup peas seasoned with diet margarine ⅓ cup mashed yellow turnips 1 cup shredded lettuce and 4 sliced small radishes mixed with low-calorie mayonnaise ½ cup canned diet fruit cocktail 1 glass skim milk

1000—Calorie Menus

No. 1

Breakfast	Small orange juice 1 slice Swiss cheese 1 piece whole-wheat toast with low-calorie jam 1 glass powdered milk
Lunch	2 hot dogs with ½ roll Tossed green salad Fresh fruit cup 1 glass powdered milk
Dinner	Small shrimp cocktail 2 ounces broiled chicken Small boiled potato with parsley Baked banana squash Fresh strawberries or canned diet fruit 1 glass powdered milk

No. 2

Breakfast
Small orange juice
1 French roll with low-calorie jam or jelly
1 ounce broiled ham
1 glass powdered milk

Lunch
2 ounces or 4 tablespoons canned salmon on bed of lettuce, with lemon or diet dressing
1 hard-boiled egg
Pickled beets
Diet cherries

Dinner
2 ounces broiled steak
Small baked potato
Summer squash
Cooked mixed-vegetable salad with diet dressing
Grapefruit-section salad
Low-calorie pudding with ¼ cup fruit
1 glass powdered milk

No. 3

Breakfast
2 stewed prunes and 2 stewed apricots
½ cup Wheatena
1 slice whole-wheat bread
1 glass powdered milk

Lunch
2-ounce slice cold roast beef
¼ cup potato salad with diet dressing
Quarter tomato and romaine
½ cantaloupe
1 glass powdered milk

Dinner
Broiled lamb chop, trimmed
Fresh asparagus
Carrots julienne
Lettuce hearts with diet dressing
1 small fresh peach
1 glass powdered milk

No. 4

Breakfast	½ sliced banana ¾ cup cornflakes 1 thin slice rye toast 1 portion farmer cheese 1 glass powdered milk
Lunch	Fresh fruit platter: sliced fresh pineapple, ½ cup berries, ¼ cup diced cantaloupe, ½ cup sliced peaches 4 tablespoons cottage cheese and 2 crackers (Melba or Ry-Krisp) 1 glass powdered milk
Dinner	2-ounce baked veal cutlet with tomato puree ¼ cup noodles String beans Tossed green salad with low-calorie dressing Small baked apple 1 diet cola

No. 5

Breakfast	½ grapefruit Omelet with 2 egg whites ½ strip crisp bacon ½ sourdough roll toasted, with low-calorie jam 1 glass powdered milk
Lunch	Tomato juice cocktail Large platter: ¼ cup crab cake, 1 hard-boiled egg, carrot curl, celery stick, and diet dressing 2 Ry-Krisps Sherbet 1 glass powdered milk

Dinner

2 ounces lean lamb fricassee
1 small carrot
1 small potato
Low-calorie dessert with ½ fresh pear
1 glass skim milk or buttermilk

No. 6

Breakfast

Sliced orange
1 poached egg with ½ piece toast
1 glass powdered milk

Lunch

½ broiled lobster, small lemon, horseradish with 1 tablespoon catsup
Mashed banana squash
String beans
Lettuce hearts with diet dressing
½ cantaloupe
1 glass powdered milk

Dinner

2-ounce slice roast beef
Small baked potato with salt
½ cup Brussels sprouts
Cole slaw with diet dressing
½ broiled peach with cinnamon and artificial sweetener
1 diet soft drink

No. 7

Breakfast

1 glass vegetable juice
2 scrambled egg whites with skim milk
1 slice toast with low-calorie jam or jelly
1 glass powdered milk

Lunch

1 broiled hamburger
Large salad with mixed greens and wine vinegar
1 slice pineapple, cubed
1 glass buttermilk

Dinner
3 ounces lean roast lamb
Generous serving lettuce and cucumbers
¼ cup cottage cheese
1 diet soft drink

No. 8

Breakfast
1 small glass grapefruit juice
⅔ cup hot oatmeal, artificially sweetened
1 glass powdered milk

Lunch
2-egg omelet with stewed or sliced tomato
¼ wedge lettuce with low-calorie dressing
1 glass powdered milk

Dinner
3 ounces baked round steak
2 celery sticks
3 spears steamed asparagus
1 boiled carrot
Low-calorie gelatin dessert
1 glass powdered milk or buttermilk

No. 9

Breakfast
4 steamed prunes
1 cup cereal with artificial sweetener
1 glass powdered milk

Lunch
4 ounces tomato juice
Chef's salad with diced cheese and ham, diet dressing
2 slices Melba toast
1 glass buttermilk

Dinner
½ skinless boiled chicken
1 cup broccoli
1 sliced tomato
1 wedge melon
1 diet cola

No. 10

Breakfast	1 glass vegetable juice 1 piece toast with cinnamon and artificial sweetener 1 glass powdered milk
Lunch	1 cup consommé ½ can tuna on bed of lettuce 1 hard-boiled egg 1 diet cola
Dinner	½ cup unsweetened melon balls 4 chicken livers with 1 slice crisp bacon 4 sliced small onions, brushed with Worcestershire sauce and broiled 1 broiled tomato ½ cup diet butterscotch pudding 1 glass powdered milk or buttermilk

1200—Calorie Menus

No. 1

Breakfast	½ sliced banana ¾ cup cornflakes 1 slice farmer cheese 1 slice whole-wheat toast with low-calorie jelly 1 glass powdered milk
Lunch	2 hot dogs ¼ cup mashed potatoes 1 cup sauerkraut Fresh fruit salad 1 small piece angel-food cake, no icing 1 diet cola
Dinner	2 ounces beef or calves' liver ½ cup noodles Cauliflower Lettuce hearts with diet dressing 2 halves diet pears 1 glass powdered milk

No. 2

Breakfast	Small glass grapefruit juice ½ cup oatmeal 1 slice whole-wheat toast with low-calorie jam or jelly 1 glass powdered milk
Lunch	Fresh fruit platter: sliced pineapple, sliced peach, sliced melon, ½ cup strawberries 4 teaspoons cottage cheese 4 Melba crackers 1 low-calorie soft drink
Dinner	3-ounce slice roast lamb ½ cup rice Broccoli Tomato aspic salad 1 cup low-calorie pudding 1 glass powdered milk

No. 3

Breakfast	3 stewed prunes 2 low-calorie pancakes 2 tablespoons low-calorie syrup 1 glass powdered milk
Lunch	2-ounce hamburger on a bun Sliced onion, sliced tomato, lettuce ¼ cup sherbet 1 glass powdered milk
Dinner	Baked fillet of sea bass Small baked potato Yellow-neck squash Tossed green salad with low-calorie dressing ¾ cup honeydew melon balls 1 diet cola

No. 4

Breakfast	¾ cup strawberries 2 Shredded Wheat biscuits 1 slice whole-wheat toast with low-calorie jam 1 glass powdered milk
Lunch	Vegetable chow mein with 2 ounces diced chicken or lean beef Sliced tomato salad ¼ cup rice Fresh pineapple chunks 1 glass buttermilk
Dinner	3-ounce baked veal chop Small baked potato ½ cup peas Fresh fruit cup or raspberry ice 1 diet cola

No. 5

Breakfast	Small orange juice ¾ cup bran flakes 1 slice rye toast with low-calorie jelly 1 glass powdered milk
Lunch	Sandwich: 2 thin slices bread with 1 thin slice cheese, 1 ounce lettuce, 1 thin slice lean ham, 1 ounce tomato, and diet mayonnaise Fresh sliced peach 1 glass powdered milk
Dinner	2 very thin slices roast turkey ¼ cup yams Fresh asparagus Tossed green salad with diet dressing ¾ cup canned melon balls 1 glass powdered milk

No. 6

Breakfast	½ grapefruit ½ cup farina 1 slice toast with low-calorie jam 1 glass powdered milk
Lunch	Platter: 2 ounces or 4 tablespoons diet tuna, 1 hard-boiled egg white, ¼ cup celery with diet dressing 1 quartered tomato ½ cup diet apricots 1 roll ½ ounce diced Swiss cheese 1 glass powdered milk or buttermilk
Dinner	2-ounce slice meat loaf Small roast potato Plain spinach with lemon seasoning Tomato salad with diet dressing ½ cup low-calorie pineapple chunks 1 glass powdered milk

No. 7

Breakfast	Sliced fresh orange Soft-boiled egg 1 slice whole-wheat toast with low-calorie jelly or margarine 1 glass powdered milk
Lunch	Open-faced cheese and crisp bacon sandwich with whole-wheat bread Relish tray of celery, carrots, cucumber slices, and pickles ½ banana 1 glass powdered milk
Dinner	1 cup clear consommé 3-ounce slice broiled liver Brussels sprouts

Watercress, onion, and radish salad with low-calorie dressing
Baked apple prepared with cinnamon and artificial sweetener
1 glass powdered milk or buttermilk

No. 8

Breakfast	Cantaloupe wedge 1 cup bran flakes with artificial sweetener 1 piece rye toast spread with diet margarine 1 glass powdered milk
Lunch	3 to 4 ounces broiled chopped meat Mixed green salad with low-calorie dressing Fresh orange sections 1 glass powdered milk or buttermilk
Dinner	2-ounce slice roast beef Small baked potato with salt ½ cup Brussels sprouts ½ grapefruit broiled with cinnamon and artificial-sweetener topping 1 diet cola

No. 9

Breakfast	1 glass vegetable juice 2 scrambled egg whites made with skim milk 1 slice toast with low-calorie jelly or jam 1 glass powdered milk
Lunch	3- to 4-ounce broiled hamburger Large mixed green salad with vinegar dressing 1 slice pineapple cubed 1 glass buttermilk

Dinner

3 ounces lean roast lamb
Generous serving lettuce and cucumbers
¼ cup cottage cheese
1 diet cola

No. 10

Breakfast

Fresh orange and grapefruit sections
Oatmeal, artificially sweetened
1 slice whole-wheat toast with diet margarine
1 glass powdered milk

Lunch

1 cup clear tomato soup
1 tablespoon cottage cheese with ½ canned pear, ½ canned diet peach, 3 steamed prunes, a dozen small grapes on lettuce bed
1 slice Melba toast
1 diet cola

Dinner

½ cup broiled shrimps with diet margarine
½ cup green peas
Curried broiled tomato
Fresh spinach with low-calorie dressing
Diet vanilla pudding
1 glass powdered milk

1500—Calorie Menus

No. 1

Breakfast

½ cup grapefruit sections
1 poached egg
1 slice whole-wheat toast with diet margarine
1 glass powdered milk

Lunch

Chef's salad: ham, cheese, tongue, tomato, and lettuce, with low-calorie dressing
2 Melba toast slices
1 dish gelatin with low-calorie topping

Dinner	3 slices roast chicken 1 riced baked potato 4 slices tomato and cucumber on lettuce leaves ½ cup diet fruit cocktail

No. 2

Breakfast	1 glass orange-grapefruit juice 1 Shredded Wheat biscuit with artificial sweetener 1 glass powdered milk
Lunch	Egg salad with low-calorie mayonnaise 3 slices tomato 1 piece fresh fruit 1 glass powdered milk
Dinner	1 ½ cups beef stew made with lean beef, carrots, onions, celery, and not more than ½ potato per serving Apple and raisin salad made with low-calorie mayonnaise 1 glass skim milk

No. 3

Breakfast	1 glass vegetable juice 1 poached egg 1 strip crisp drained bacon 1 slice whole-wheat toast 1 glass powdered milk
Lunch	1 ground chicken, egg, and onion patty ½ cup noodles with 2 tablespoons cheese sauce ½ cup spinach seasoned with vinegar 2 canned diet pear halves 1 glass skim milk

Dinner
6 large broiled scallops
¾ cup green beans and mushrooms
1 small boiled potato
⅔ cup orange sections and fresh pitted cherries
1 diet cola

No. 4

Breakfast
½ cantaloupe
1 soft-boiled egg
1 slice cracked-wheat toast with diet margarine
1 glass powdered milk

Lunch
4 medium-size fish sticks with lemon, pickle, and diet mayonnasie
Cole slaw with diet mayonnaise
½ cup fresh fruit
1 diet cola

Dinner
1 slice (3 ounces) London broil
½ cup cooked diced beets, ½ cup cooked green beans seasoned with vinegar
½ cup rice
1 scoop sherbet
1 glass skim milk

No. 5

Breakfast
1 glass vegetable juice
French toast, oven-baked with egg whites, sweetened with cinnamon
1 glass powdered milk

Lunch
Clear consommé
Tuna salad made with diet mayonnaise
Baked apple seasoned with cinnamon and artificial sweetener
1 diet cola

Dinner

1 cup veal stew with carrots, onions, and 1 small boiled potato
1 medium tomato, sliced, sprinkled with chopped dill
Wedge of lettuce with low-calorie dressing
1 glass powdered milk

No. 6

Breakfast

1 cup fresh fruit
1 scrambled egg
1 slice whole-wheat toast, diet margarine
1 glass powdered milk

Lunch

1 cup clear vegetable soup (dried)
1 grilled lamb patty
½ cup noodles
½ tomato sliced on lettuce with lemon seasoning
1 glass powdered milk

Dinner

2 large broiled lamb chops with 1 slice toast
½ cup cooked green beans
1 small boiled potato with diet margarine, parsley
½ cup cooked mushrooms
1 cup diet vanilla pudding, ½ banana sliced
1 diet cola

No. 7

Breakfast

½ grapefruit
1 poached egg
½ bun with low-calorie jelly or jam
1 glass powdered milk

Lunch

1 cup tomato soup
1 hot dog with ½ roll and 1 teaspoon mustard
1 large dill pickle
½ cup fruit gelatin
1 glass skim milk

Dinner

1 small glass low-calorie cranberry juice
1 3-inch-square poached salmon
6 spears steamed asparagus with low-calorie margarine
2 tablespoons cottage cheese
2-tomato salad mold
1 diet cola

No. 8

Breakfast

½ small grapefruit
1 fried egg, drained
1 slice whole-wheat toast with diet margarine
1 glass powdered milk

Lunch

1 cup roast beef hash
2 tablespoons chili sauce
½ cup shredded carrots, ¼ cup minced celery mixed with 1 tablespoon diet mayonnaise
1 small apple
1 glass skim milk or buttermilk

Dinner

1 broiled medium club steak, fat trimmed
½ cup cooked spinach with hard-boiled egg
½ cucumber sliced with 1 tablespoon chopped onion, flavored with vinegar
1 diet cola

No. 9

Breakfast

1 cup fresh melon balls
Eggnog made with 1 glass skim milk, artificial sweetener, and nutmeg to taste

Lunch

2 medium slices liverwurst
Lettuce and tomato salad with diet dressing
2 tablespoons cottage cheese with 4 steamed prunes
1 glass powdered milk

Dinner
6 medium broiled shrimps with lemon seasoning
½ cup rice with low-calorie curry
½ cup cole slaw with diet mayonnaise
1 small piece angel cake, no icing
1 diet cola

No. 10

Breakfast
1 cup grapefruit and orange sections
1 scrambled egg
1 piece whole-wheat toast with diet margarine
1 glass powdered milk

Lunch
1 cup chicken noodle soup (dried pack)
1 toasted open sandwich: 1 slice cheese on rye bread topped with 1 slice crisp bacon
3 canned diet apricots
1 glass powdered milk

Dinner
1 ½ cups beef stew made with lean beef, carrots, onion, and not more than 1 small potato per serving
1 mixed salad with lemon seasoning
1 cup vanilla diet pudding

No. 11

Breakfast
1 glass orange juice
2 eggs scrambled with 2 tablespoons buttermilk
1 glass powdered milk

Lunch
Clear consommé
½ cup tuna salad made with diet mayonnaise
1 diet cola

Dinner	2 lamb chops, trimmed ½ cup cooked green beans 1 small boiled potato, diet margarine, parsley ½ cup cooked mushrooms 1 cup sherbet

No. 12

Breakfast	¼ melon in season, or frozen melon balls Eggnog made with skim milk, nutmeg, artificial sweetener
Lunch	2 medium slices liverwurst Lettuce and tomato salad with low-calorie dressing 2 tablespoons cottage cheese with 4 steamed prunes 1 diet cola
Dinner	6 medium broiled shrimps with lemon seasoning ½ cup rice with low-calorie curry ½ cup cole slaw with diet mayonnaise 1 cup diet gelatin with fruit 1 glass powdered milk

No. 13

Breakfast	½ grapefruit 1 boiled egg 1 roll with diet jam 1 glass powdered milk
Lunch	1 slice ham 1 slice cheese 3 slices tomato ¼ dill pickle 1 cup sherbet 1 glass powdered milk

Dinner
1 lamb chop, fat trimmed
1 broiled tomato
1 small riced potato
Carrots and celery sticks
1 glass powdered milk

1500 to 2000—Calorie Menus

No. 1—1625 Calories

Breakfast
1 small glass orange juice
2 baked eggs
1 piece whole-wheat toast, diet margarine
1 glass powdered milk

Lunch
1 5-inch piece broiled flounder with diet tartar sauce (made with diet mayonnaise, pickle, lemon)
½ cup green peas
½ cup spinach creamed with diet white sauce
1 cup fresh or diet cherries
1 glass powdered milk

Dinner
Clear consommé
4 thin slices chicken
½ cup macaroni
½ cup green beans
1 small piece un-iced sponge cake
1 diet cola

No. 2—1900 Calories

Breakfast
1 glass vegetable juice
1 Shredded Wheat biscuit artificially sweetened, topped with ½ banana
1 cup powdered milk

Lunch
1 cup vegetable soup (dried)
Egg salad made with diet mayonnaise
Lettuce and tomato wedges
½ cup low-calorie chocolate pudding
1 glass powdered milk

Dinner
2 broiled hamburger patties
1 baked potato
½ cup okra
1 mixed green salad with lemon seasoning
2 fresh plums or 1 pear
1 slice whole-wheat bread with diet margarine
1 diet cola

No. 3—1850 Calories

Breakfast
½ grapefruit
1 waffle with low-calorie syrup
1 glass powdered milk

Lunch
1 cup Manhattan clam chowder
2 thin slices ham
½ cup macaroni salad with pickles and diet mayonnaise
½ cup Italian green beans
1 diet cola

Dinner
4 chicken livers
½ cup rice
½ cup Brussels sprouts
1 wedge lettuce with diet dressing
1 glass powdered milk

No. 4—1800 Calories

Breakfast
Sliced orange
2 scrambled eggs
1 slice Canadian bacon
½ toasted roll with diet jelly or jam
1 glass powdered milk

Lunch
Crabmeat salad: ½ cup crabmeat, 1 hard-cooked egg, 3 green onions, 3 radishes, 1 tablespoon diet Russian dressing
1 slice whole-wheat bread with diet margarine
1 diet cola

Dinner
- 1 thin slice baked canned ham
- ¾ cup buttered green beans and mushrooms
- ½ cup mashed squash
- Celery and carrot strips
- Sherbet with 2 spoons canned diet berries
- 1 glass powdered milk

No. 5—1800 Calories

Breakfast
- Orange-grapefruit juice
- 1 poached egg
- 1 slice whole-wheat toast with low-calorie jelly
- 1 glass powdered milk

Lunch
- ¾ cup cream of tomato soup
- Open chicken sandwich with 2 ounces diet dressing and 1 slice canned, boned chicken on whole-wheat bread
- Baked apple sweetened with cinnamon and sugar substitute
- 1 diet cola

Dinner
- New England boiled dinner: 1 slice corned beef, 3 small canned potatoes, 1 cabbage wedge, and 1 medium-sized carrot
- 1 corn stick with diet margarine
- 4 medium diet apricot halves
- 1 glass powdered milk or buttermilk

No. 6—1800 Calories

Breakfast
- ½ cantaloupe
- ½ cup bran flakes with sugar substitute
- 1 slice toasted raisin bread with diet margarine
- 1 glass powdered milk

Lunch
1 frankfurter
¾ cup mashed potatoes made with skim milk
Sauerkraut
Carrot sticks
1 slice whole-wheat toast with low-calorie jam
2 peach halves
1 diet cola

Dinner
3 ounces broiled sirloin, trimmed
1 stalk broccoli
½ cup sweet potatoes
3 slices tomato and lettuce with low-calorie French dressing
1 hard roll with diet jam
½ cup baked custard
1 glass powdered milk

No. 7—1850 Calories

Breakfast
Small orange juice
2 soft-cooked eggs
Corn muffin with diet margarine
1 glass powdered milk

Lunch
Clear consommé
Salmon salad plate: ½ cup canned salmon, ½ cup cottage cheese, and 1 medium tomato
1 melba toast
1 diet cola

Dinner
¼ broiled chicken
½ cup green beans
1 ear corn with diet margarine
½ cup cole slaw
1 slice angel cake, no icing
1 glass powdered milk

No. 8—1800 Calories

Breakfast
3 figs in syrup
2 pancakes with low-calorie syrup
1 glass powdered milk

Lunch
½ cup cream of pea soup
½ broiled lobster
½ cup mashed banana squash
6 Brussels sprouts
1 square low-calorie gelatin
1 diet cola

Dinner
Baked veal chop, trimmed
½ cup tomatoes boiled with ½ cup noodles, ½ cup chopped onion, 1 tablespoon catsup, and 1 teaspoon chopped green pepper
½ cup shredded carrots with raisins and diet dressing
3 large ladyfingers
1 glass powdered milk

No. 9—1900 Calories

Breakfast
1 cup orange sections
⅔ cup hot cereal
1 ounce Polish sausage
1 slice whole-wheat toast with diet jam
1 glass powdered milk

Lunch
1 cup vegetable soup
3 diet crackers
2-egg Western omelet with green pepper, green onion, and bits of ham
1 slice pineapple with 2 tablespoons cottage cheese
1 glass powdered milk

Dinner
2 slices broiled beef liver
½ cup frozen lima beans
½ cup Harvard beets
Tossed green salad with diet dressing
Raspberry sherbet
1 hard roll with diet margarine
1 diet cola

No. 10—1950 Calories

Breakfast
1 glass orange-grapefruit juice
1 soft-cooked egg
1 slice whole-wheat toast with diet margarine
1 glass powdered milk

Lunch
Clear consommé
Grilled open cheese and bacon sandwich: 1 slice American cheese, 1 bacon strip
Relish tray: celery, carrots, radishes, 2 olives
1 banana with 1 teaspoon peanut butter, 1 teaspoon low-calorie dressing
1 glass powdered milk

Dinner
2 thin slices rib roast
1 potato, riced
Sliced carrots braised with bouillon cube and water
Watercress, onion and radish salad with diet French dressing
2 tablespoons cottage cheese
1 slice rye bread
1 baked apple with cinnamon and sugar substitute

7

Seven-Day Diet Menu

Variety is not only the spice of life, it's the secret of success with a diet. Keeping your child interested in low-calorie food is going to require all your ingenuity and skill as a cook.

In order to make sure that your portion control is exact, serve food in the kitchen. Those members of the family who need to gain weight can have bigger helpings of everything. One trick I have learned about serving food to overweight children is to use a plate a little bit smaller than everyone else's. They will seldom notice the difference, and you can cover their plates with food so it looks as though they are getting as much as the rest of the family.

If the smaller plate trick does not work, try covering as much of the plate as possible by garnishing the service with lettuce, raw vegetables, and relishes. The meal will look appealing as well as generous.

The following seven-day, well-balanced diet, based on 1,200

calories a day, should prove helpful as a guide to making up a similar diet tailored to your child's daily caloric needs.

First Day

Breakfast	Orange juice (4 ounces) Poached eggs (2) Toast (1 slice) Butter or margarine (1 pat) Powdered milk (if desired)
Lunch	Braised lamb chop (3 ounces) Broccoli (½ cup) Lettuce-tomato salad Milk, nonfat (1 cup)
Dinner	Blade pot roast (4 ounces) Green beans (½ cup) Butter or margarine (1 pat) Peaches, water-packed or fresh without sugar (½ cup) Milk, nonfat (1 cup) Coffee or tea (if desired)

NOTE: Half the pat of butter on the dinner menu could be used on broccoli at lunch and the other on beans at dinner.

In this and the following menus, the cup of nonfat milk at dinner can be used later for bedtime snack if desired.

Second Day

Breakfast	Grapefruit (½) Soft-cooked eggs (2) Toast (1 slice) Butter or margarine (1 pat) Powdered milk (if desired)
Lunch	Ground beef patty (3 ounces) Beets (½ cup) Mayonnaise (1 tablespoon) Cole slaw (½ cup) Milk, nonfat (1 cup)

Dinner	Tomato juice (3 ounces) Baked salmon or baked ham (4 ounces) Spinach (½ cup) Butter or margarine (1 pat) Carrot sticks (½ carrot) Coffee or tea (if desired) Milk, nonfat (1 cup)

Third Day

Breakfast	Orange slices Poached eggs (2) Toast (1 slice) Butter or margarine (1 pat) Coffee or tea (if desired)
Lunch	Fried liver (4 ounces) with bacon (2 slices) Green peas (½ cup) Lettuce wedge (1/6 head) French dressing (1 tablespoon) Milk, nonfat (1 cup) Coffee or tea (if desired)
Dinner	Roast leg of lamb (4 ounces) Carrots (½ cup) Butter or margarine (1 pat) Cabbage-pineapple salad (½ cup) Milk, nonfat (1 cup) Coffee or tea (if desired)

Fourth Day

Breakfast	Orange juice (4 ounces) Soft-cooked eggs (2) Toast (1 slice) Butter or margarine (1 pat) Coffee or tea (if desired)

Lunch
Luncheon meat salad (3 ounces meat with ¼ cup chopped celery and green pepper)
Stewed tomatoes (½ cup)
Milk, nonfat (1 cup)
Coffee or tea (if desired)

Dinner
Smoked shoulder butt (4 ounces)
Cabbage (½ cup)
Butter or margarine (1 pat)
Grapefruit sections, unsweetened or fresh without sugar (½ cup)
Milk, nonfat (1 cup)
Coffee or tea (if desired)

Fifth Day

Breakfast
Grapefruit juice (4 ounces)
Cereal, unsweetened (1 cup) with milk, nonfat (¼ cup)
Toast (1 slice)
Butter or margarine (1 pat)
Coffee or tea (if desired)

Lunch
Tomato juice (3 ounces)
Beef brisket (3 ounces)
Green beans (½ cup)
Lettuce wedge (1/6 head)
Milk, nonfat (1 cup)
Coffee or tea (if desired)

Dinner
Ground beef patty (4 ounces)
Cauliflower (½ cup)
Butter or margarine (1 pat)
Carrot sticks (½ carrot)
Vanilla ice cream (¼ pint)
Milk, nonfat (1 cup)
Coffee or tea (if desired)

Sixth Day

Breakfast	Orange juice (4 ounces) Canadian-style bacon (3 slices) Toast (1 slice) Butter or margarine (1 pat) Coffee or tea (if desired)
Lunch	Pork chop (3 ounces) Squash (½ cup) Apple-celery salad on lettuce (⅓ cup chopped apple, ¼ cup chopped celery) Milk, nonfat (1 cup) Coffee or tea (if desired)
Dinner	Tomato juice (2 ounces) Roast beef (4 ounces) Wax beans (½ cup) Butter or margarine (1 pat) Celery sticks Milk, nonfat (1 cup) Coffee or tea (if desired)

Seventh Day

Breakfast	Grapefruit sections (½ cup) Scrambled eggs (2) Toast (1 slice) Butter or margarine (1 pat) Coffee or tea (if desired)
Lunch	Sirloin steak (3 ounces) Boiled onions (½ cup) Cottage cheese and peach salad Milk, nonfat (1 cup) Coffee or tea (if desired)

Dinner

Roast turkey or roast pork loin (4 ounces)
Carrots (½ cup)
Butter or margarine (1 pat)
Sliced tomato (small)
Diet French dressing (½ tablespoon)
Milk, nonfat (1 cup)
Coffee or tea (if desired)

8

Carry-Out Lunches

For the dieting child, lunchtime can be the cruelest hour of the day. Few school lunchrooms make any provision for the child who is counting his calories; even the salad plates contain mayonnaise and carbohydrates.

Here are some lunches your child can take to school or to outings with his friends. These lunches will enable him to look forward to meals away from home as much as he does to those around the family table.

For the fruit and cooked vegetables in these lunches, you will need plastic containers with lids that lock securely. You will find that plastic bags are excellent for sandwiches, and a thermos is very useful for hot bouillon and low-calorie soups on cold days and for skim milk plus a little low-calorie sweetener on hot days.

School Lunch No. 1

Ripe Olive and Celery Sandwich—235 Calories

Dice 1 stalk celery, mince 4 ripe olives, and blend with 1 teaspoon relish. Spread between 2 slices low-calorie brown bread along with a leaf of lettuce.

⅔ cup raw cauliflower
½ cup fresh cherries
1 can diet cola—or add 85 calories for skim milk

School Lunch No. 2

Dried Bacon and Celery Sandwich—235 calories

Fry 2 slices lean bacon until crisp. Drain thoroughly on absorbent paper and crumble. Dice ½ stalk celery and mix with bacon and 1 teaspoon relish. Spread on low-calorie brown bread along with slice of lettuce.

8 cucumber slices
½ cup fresh berries or canned diet fruit
1 can diet cola—or add 85 calories for skim milk

School Lunch No. 3

Cottage Cheese and Raw Vegetable Sandwich—235 calories

Combine 2 tablespoons cottage cheese with 2 tablespoons raw peas, 2 tablespoons grated carrot, and ¼ teaspoon onion salt. Spread between 2 slices low-calorie brown bread.

1 medium tomato
3 prunes
1 can diet cola—or add 85 calories for skim milk

School Lunch No. 4

Shrimp and Chopped Chive Sandwich—250 calories

Dice ⅓ cup cooked shrimps. Blend with 1 teaspoon relish, ½ teaspoon chopped chives, and 1 teaspoon chili sauce. Spread mixture on low-calorie brown bread along with slice of lettuce.

2 large celery stalks
1 medium banana
1 can diet cola—or add 85 calories for skim milk

School Lunch No. 5

Chopped Liver and Relish Sandwich—240 calories

Sauté 1 piece calves' liver 1 ½ inches square in ⅓ teaspoon butter. Chop finely. Mix with 1 teaspoon India relish and 1 teaspoon diet mayonnaise. Spread between two slices low-calorie brown bread along with leaf of lettuce.

Carrot strips
2 fresh plums
1 can diet cola—or add 85 calories for skim milk

School Lunch No. 6

Diced Meat and Cole Slaw Sandwich—230 calories

Dice finely 1 ounce cooked meat. Chop finely ¼ cup cabbage. Mix both with 1 teaspoon relish and 1 teaspoon chili sauce. Spread between 2 slices low-calorie brown bread.

2 stalks celery
1 slice pineapple
1 can diet cola—or add 85 calories for skim milk

School Lunch No. 7

Dieter's Club Sandwich—420 calories

Place 1 slice each boiled ham and Swiss cheese along with lettuce leaf and green pepper strips on white bread. Lightly spread with diet margarine.

3 dried apricots
1 raw carrot
1 can diet cola—or add 85 calories for skim milk

School Lunch No. 8

480 calories

1 chicken drumstick, broiled or roasted
1 cup chilled green beans in 2 tablespoons diet dressing
1 small orange
2 diet cookies
1 diet cola

School Lunch No. 9

500 calories

Small thermos tomato soup
Open cheese sandwich made with 1 slice white bread, 2 slices American cheese, and 1 tablespoon pickle relish
1 small apple
1 can diet cola—or add 85 calories for skim milk

School Lunch No. 10

350 calories

Open roast sandwich made with 1 slice white bread lightly spread with relish, 1 slice beef, lamb, pork, or veal
½ cucumber
3 radishes
1 cup applesauce
1 can diet cola—or add 85 calories for skim milk

School Lunch No. 11

400 calories

Thermos of cream of vegetable soup with ⅓ cup cooked chicken added.
1 tomato
1 container low-calorie dessert
1 can diet cola—or add 85 calories for skim milk

School Lunch No. 12

400 calories

2 deviled eggs made with pickle relish
½ carrot
3 celery stalks
1 small roll, lightly spread with diet margarine
1 bunch seedless grapes
1 can diet cola—or add 85 calories for skim milk

9

Notes on Nutrition

Make sure your child has one or two tablespoons of fat—butter, margarine or oil—every day. I know it may sound ridiculous to give fat to a child who is trying to lose weight, but fat is necessary for growth. Fat contains lecithin and linoleic acid that help the body change sugar to body fat more slowly and reduce the amount of water held by the tissues. A small amount of fat also helps produce those signposts of good health—rosy cheeks.

A good diet does not eliminate all fattening foods, but it does control the calorie intake and food portions of the person who wants to lose weight. I have seen cases in which parents were so concerned about counting calories they forgot that food has nutritional value, too. Obsessed by the idea of foods being fattening, they became blinded to nutritional needs and fed their children into ill health.

It's still difficult for some parents to accept that the chubby little boy who keeps stuffing himself may actually be undernourished. Those goodies he devours have little or no food value.

Even though his stomach always feels bloated and the fat continues to spread over his frame, the poor child may actually be starving—from a nutritional point of view. If a child's weight-loss program is to work, his diet must still afford him enough food and vitamins to maintain his energy and health.

Food values are an old subject, but I want to stress them again because I think most people tend to forget about the nutritional value of food when they start counting calories. These are facts that you should keep in mind when making up weekly menus.

Protein is the essential fuel of all living organisms. An adult requires about 70 grams of protein just to replace worn-out tissues; but an adolescent whose body is still growing needs 180 grams. Some food sources of protein are better than others because they also contain amino acids, which are vital to the building of body tissues. A third of your child's protein should come from poultry, meat, and fish; the remainder from eggs or some form of milk. Eggs also contain lecithin and linoleic acids, which give elasticity to muscles.

When you begin to keep a closer watch on how much protein you are serving, you may notice that your youngster seems somewhat more stable emotionally. Instead of quick bursts of energy that come when some sweet or carbohydrate raises the blood-sugar level, there is a steady flow of energy as the protein is consumed. A proper intake of protein will help your child get off the physical and emotional roller-coaster ride that comes from eating sweets which raise the blood sugar dramatically, give the child an emotional "high," and then plunge him into a depressing "low" again once the body has used up all the energy.

Carbohydrates are the most plentiful sources of energy. Almost 50 percent of the calories people consume come from carbohydrates. On the other hand, carbohydrates are one of the leading sources of fat in overweight children.

Carbohydrates are essential to the daily business of living. Something as untaxing as a smile requires the kind of energy that we get from them. The trick in doling out carbohydrates is to achieve a proper balance. And this is very hard to do. It's virtually impossible to say what a child's daily intake of carbohydrates should be. Every child is different and has his own energy needs.

The best advice I can offer is to keep a watchful eye on your child and be ready to act if he seems listless and overtired. Use common sense when serving his food. A heaping helping of mashed potatoes is obviously too much, yet no potatoes would deprive your child of an important source of energy. Fortunately, most mothers seem to develop a "feel" for the right amount of carbohydrates for their child, based upon a combination of instinct and sharp observation.

Milk has been so overemphasized as a food for children that adolescents often rebel against it as part of the trappings of childhood. But milk remains one of the best possible foods and for a dieting child, it's essential.

You should try to get your youngster to drink at least two glasses of skim or powdered milk every day. If he balks at this amount, give him cottage cheese or yogurt. Plain vanilla yogurt may be "doctored" with low-calorie flavorings to appeal to your child's taste.

Milk is rich in protein and in vitamins C and A, which happen to be the vitamins most often lacking in the American diet. Milk also contains calcium, a mineral necessary for building bones.

One of the welcome side effects of serving milk may be a more emotionally stable teen-ager. A lack of calcium in the diet often causes many teen-agers to become irritable and restless.

Minerals are needed in amounts which seem so small they are hardly worth the worry. Yet if they aren't in our diet, we find ourselves beset with all kinds of health problems.

Iron is needed to build healthy red blood; without it some form of anemia develops. Leafy vegetables, eggs, and cereal products are the best sources of iron.

Iodine is commonly found in iodized salt and seafood. Goiter, a swelling of the thyroid gland on the neck, is caused by a lack of iodine. This disease has virtually disappeared now that iodized salt is on the market.

Many people have begun to experiment with salt-free diets and with salt to which iodine has not been added, but it should be remembered that iodine is still essential to the diet.

Vitamins are needed daily, although in small amounts, to maintain health and promote growth.

Vitamin A primarily builds resistance to disease, but is often called the "cosmetic" vitamin because it improves the complexion, hair, and eyes. It is commonly found in beef, liver, halibut, eggs, dairy products, and yellow vegetables.

Vitamin B_1 helps stabilize emotions while its mate,

Vitamin B_2 prevents eye problems and is helpful to the child with oily skin and hair. Both B vitamins are found in liver, eggs, and whole-grain breads and cereals.

Vitamin B_6 is often called the "morale" vitamin because it combats depression. It is found in liver, eggs, and whole-grain cereals.

Vitamin C has received considerable publicity recently as a kind of miracle drug for combating colds. I don't want to get involved in the controversy over whether vitamin C actually works wonders against a cold once you have caught one, but it has been long recognized for its power to help build up one's resistance to the common cold. Citrus fruits and vegetables are still the best sources of vitamin C.

Vitamin D is the famous "sunshine" vitamin. It helps children absorb minerals that build strong bones. Lack of vitamin D causes rickets, an appalling disease that results in bent and brittle bones. We rarely see a case of rickets today because of the abundance of vitamin supplements and the knowledge that vitamin D is found in fish, liver, egg yolk, and animal fats.

10

Hamburger Delights for Young Dieters

Ask most children what their favorite food is and chances are they will say hamburgers or hot dogs. For the parent trying to help a child lose weight, hamburgers, specially prepared, can be a great ally. This chapter includes a half dozen recipes for ground meat that will add great variety to your menu.

In some cases, I have specified veal instead of beef. Veal, a white, bland meat from young calves, has proven itself a great aid to dieters. It contains only one quarter the amount of cholesterol found in beef. A three-ounce serving of veal has 185 calories compared to 380 calories in a three-ounce serving of roast beef. So whenever possible, try to substitute veal for beef.

When using ground beef, always avoid preground hamburgers. Almost invariably, preground beef is rich in calories.

Ground round is the lowest in fat content, but it's also the most expensive. In addition it tends to dry out quickly.

Ground chuck meat, on the other hand, is less expensive and juicier than ground round. And it tastes better.

Broiled Hamburger

This is the standard hamburger dressed up with a few spices.

1 pound ground meat
1 level dessert spoon of prepared mustard
2 heaping tablespoons of ketchup or chili sauce
1 egg
¾ cup ice cold water
1 small onion, well grated
Salt and pepper to taste

Mix all the ingredients together in a large bowl. Shape into six patties. Broil for 10 to 15 minutes.

Calories per hamburger: 185
Makes 6 portions

Supreme Relish for Hamburgers

You can whip up a batch of this sweet and pungent relish and keep it on hand for weeks.

1 cup chopped uncooked onion
1 cup chopped uncooked green pepper
1 cup chopped uncooked sweet red pepper
2 tablespoons margarine
2 tablespoons cooking oil
3 tablespoons Worcestershire sauce
1 tablespoon lemon juice
¾ cup tomato ketchup
¾ cup brown sugar
1 teaspoon salt
12 drops hot sauce or Tabasco sauce
10 whole cloves
1 stick cinnamon
¼ teaspoon ground cloves

In an enamel skillet, cook onion and red and green peppers in margarine and cooking oil until they are soft but not brown.

Add the rest of the ingredients and cook for three minutes over a medium heat. Keep tasting until you are satisfied they are well blended.

The relish can be served hot or stored in the refrigerator. Calories per tablespoon of relish: 25

Hong Kong Hamburgers

Chinese food is always popular with children and particularly with teen-agers. These Chinese-style hamburgers can be served on buns or on plates with vegetables. Mixed with rice and canned bean sprouts, you can use them as the heart of an "instant chop suey."

1½ pounds ground veal
¼ cup canned water chestnuts, finely chopped
1 teaspoon ginger
2 tablespoons soy sauce
1 teaspoon black pepper
1 teaspoon peanut oil

Combine veal, water chestnuts, ginger, soy sauce, and black pepper in a mixing bowl. Shape into four patties.

Heat peanut oil until it just begins to smoke. Drop patties in and cook until the outside is brown. Reduce heat and cook until desired doneness.

Calories per patty: 180
Makes 4 portions

Hamburgers, Mrs. Mason Special

I concocted these for my boys and girls at Camp Tahoe and Camp Stanley. I have added liver to these hamburgers, although liver probably heads the food "hate-list" for most children. But it is an excellent source of protein and minerals. When mixed with hamburger, my campers don't even notice it's there.

I would advise you not to say anything to your family about mixing liver with the hamburger. If there aren't any complaints, you can add it to hamburger in other recipes and thereby increase the food value.

You may be surprised to learn that this recipe calls for a half teaspoon of butter with each patty. But, as I explained earlier, a small amount of fat is necessary for good health. In this case, the butter should be part of the day's fat content.

1½ pounds ground round beef
½ pound liver
4 tablespoons minced onion
3 tablespoons chopped carrot
3 tablespoons chopped celery
3 tablespoons chopped parsley
1 tablespoon vegetable oil
2 tablespoons butter
1 teaspoon Tabasco sauce
1 tablespoon Worcestershire sauce
1 tablespoon lemon juice

Sauté the onion and liver until the onions are soft, and the liver is lightly done. (Don't let the meat harden on the outside.)

Put the liver and onions through the meat grinder at the same time. In a large mixing bowl, thoroughly mix the liver, beef, and all the chopped vegetables except the parsley. Shape into patties and sprinkle each side with some chopped parsley. With the heel of your hand, gently press the parsley into the meat patties and let stand for 30 minutes.

For a rare hamburger, cook in oil for 30 seconds over high heat, and then over medium heat for an additional minute. (Cook longer at medium heat to preferred doneness.)

Place ½ teaspoon butter on each patty. Add Tabasco, Worcestershire, and lemon juice to the pan. When butter has melted, remove patties from the pan and place on a heated platter. Lower heat. Using a wire wisk, swirl the sauce in the pan. Pour it over the patties and serve.

Calories per serving: 200
Makes 6 portions

Chili Con Carne

Chili is a particular favorite among teen-agers. Unfortunately, most store-bought or restaurant chilies are filled with calories and spices. This recipe will allow you to prepare a delicious, low-calorie chili at home. And it is an excellent dish to serve at young peoples' parties; guests will never know your child is on a diet.

1 tablespoon salad oil
1 clove garlic, thinly sliced

1 cup chopped onion
2 cups sliced celery
½ cup chopped green pepper
1 pound ground round beef
¼ pound liver, ground or minced
1 pound canned kidney beans, drained
1 pound canned tomatoes
½ teaspoon salt
1½ teaspoons chili powder

In salad oil, in a 4-quart kettle, sauté garlic, onion, celery, and green pepper until onion is light brown. Add beef and liver and cook until the meat is browned. Stir in kidney beans, tomatoes, salt, and chili powder. Simmer mixture at least 45 minutes to blend flavors.

This recipe can be prepared in advance and then cooled in a refrigerator. Heat slowly about 20 minutes before serving time. (If you reheat and you prefer your chili hot, stir in a little fresh chili powder.)

Calories per portion: 155
Makes 8 portions

Sweet and Sour Stuffed Cabbage

Here is another dish that can be served at a party or on a festive occasion. It will lend an exotic touch to your dinner table.

1 small head cabbage
1 pound ground round beef
¼ pound liver
1 small onion, finely chopped
¼ cup bread crumbs
½ teaspoon salt
1 onion, thinly sliced
1 medium-sized carrot, sliced
1 cup beef consommé
1 cup canned tomatoes
1 tablespoon lemon juice
1 tablespoon brown sugar
1 teaspoon salt

Cut out core of the cabbage. Place the cabbage in a saucepan of boiling water. Simmer for five minutes. Remove from water and carefully remove eight outer leaves. Cut about four slices from the remaining cabbage to use in recipe. (Leftover cabbage may be used in another meal.)

Sauté liver and chopped onion until both are lightly done. Put through grinder together.

In a mixing bowl, combine beef, liver, onion, bread crumbs, water, and ½ teaspoon salt. Fill each cabbage leaf with ¼ cup of the meat filling. Roll up tight and fasten with toothpick. Place cabbage rolls in deep saucepan, folded side down; add sliced cabbage, sliced onion, carrot, and then consommé.

Cook over low heat for 1 hour, stirring occasionally. Add tomatoes, lemon juice, brown sugar, and 1 teaspoon salt. Simmer gently for 15 minutes, then remove from heat and serve.

Calories per serving: 240

Makes 6 servings

11

Low-Calorie Gourmet Delights

Don't throw away your cookbook when you start diet cooking. Look over your favorite recipes and check the ingredients against the calorie counter. See if you can cut down calories or switch ingredients. With a few judicious substitutions, you probably can still prepare your favorite recipes. Gourmet cooking for the dieter is a matter of combining imagination with mathematics.

Tuna Antipasto

Fish is an excellent source of protein and is lower in calories than meat. In this country, however, many children have been raised to eat meat and ignore fish. But most youngsters don't consider tuna to be fish—after all, it doesn't look or smell like fish, and it comes in a can.

Tuna comes packed in water or oil. Try to purchase the water pack. If you buy the other, drain the fish thoroughly before using.

One of the simplest tuna dishes I know makes an excellent and filling hors d'oeuvre. You will also find that tuna is the main ingredient in many casserole dishes.

1 6-ounce can tuna
Radishes, celery, and fennel
Lettuce leaves

Turn tuna onto bed of lettuce. Garnish with radishes, celery, and fennel.

Season with lemon or vinegar and salt and pepper to taste. Sprinkle with paprika.

Calories per 3-ounce serving: 180

Makes 4 servings

Shrimps with Rice, Italian Style

Shrimps are an excellent source of protein, yet they are low in calories.

1 pound cooked shrimps
1 tablespoon cooking oil
⅓ cup sliced onion
½ cup diced celery
2 cups canned tomatoes
1 tablespoon chopped sweet basil
Salt and pepper to taste

To cook shrimps, simmer in water until pink. Be careful not to let water boil.

Sauté onion and celery in oil until tender. Add tomatoes, basil, salt and pepper. Simmer for 20 minutes.

Add cooked clean shrimps and cover. Cook about five minutes longer. Serve over boiled rice.

Calories per 3-ounce serving: 170

Makes 4 servings

Chicken Cacciatore

This is a restaurant specialty that you can make quickly and easily at home. It will still any resentment other family members may harbor about sharing the "diet food" of the child who is trying to lose weight.

1 chicken, approximately 2 pounds, cut up for frying
2 medium onions, sliced
1 clove garlic, finely chopped
1 green pepper, seeded and cut into slices
1 cup canned tomatoes
1 cup sliced mushrooms
Salt and pepper to taste

Season chicken with salt and pepper. Brown on all sides in skillet. If you use a teflon skillet, no oil is needed.

Add garlic, green pepper, onions, and tomatoes. Cover and simmer slowly for 40 minutes. Add mushrooms and simmer until mushrooms and chicken are tender.

Calories per 3-ounce serving: 150

Makes 6 servings

Cinnamon Toast

This traditional American dish can be served as the heart of a special breakfast treat, as a midmorning or a midafternoon snack, or as a dessert to top off a light meal.

1 slice white bread
1 teaspoon oil or butter
¼ teaspoon sugar
¾ teaspoon cinnamon

Toast bread. Spread one side of slice with oil or butter. Mix sugar and cinnamon together and sprinkle over the toast.

Calories per slice: 110

Blintzes with Mock Sour Cream

Generally, these cheese pancakes are considered a traditional Jewish dish, but they can be found in different versions in many European countries. This recipe calls for a cheese filling, but a fruit filling can be substituted.

1 cup flour
3 teaspoons baking powder
2 tablespoons sugar
½ teaspoon salt

2 whole eggs, beaten
1¼ cups whole milk
3 tablespoons butter, shortening, or oil

Mix flour, baking powder, sugar, and salt. Beat eggs, then add milk and shortening to them (liquify shortening if you are not using oil). Stir in flour mixture and blend until smooth. Let the mixture rest for about an hour.

Lightly oil a small frying pan and heat. Pour in batter and tilt it from side to side until the whole pan is thinly coated. Brown pancake on one side and turn over. Cook the other side lightly but do not brown. Lay pancakes out flat, ready for filling.

Filling

Combine 1 lightly beaten egg with 1 cup creamed cottage cheese, 1 tablespoon sugar, and a pinch of cinnamon.

Spread brown side of pancake with the filling, then roll. Return rolled blintzes to the frying pan for final browning.

Calories per blintze: 65

Makes 8 blintzes

Mock Sour Cream

This low-calorie substitute for sour cream tastes as good as the real thing, and it can be used whenever sour cream is required. It's particularly tasty served with blintzes.

3 tablespoons lemon juice
3 tablespoons liquid skim milk or fat-free buttermilk
8 ounces cottage cheese

Put lemon juice and milk in blender. Blend at low speed and add cottage cheese gradually. Then blend a few minutes at high speed. (If cream becomes too thick on standing, thin it with skim or fat-free buttermilk to desired consistency.)

Calories per ounce: 30

Lamb Curry

Curries originated in India. However, during the period when India was part of the British Empire, the English became so fond of lamb curry that now it might be considered an English dish.

If your family likes chili, they should like lamb curry. Exercise extreme caution, if you happen to use an English or Indian curry. Indian curry is only slightly cooler than Tabasco sauce, and you will need very little to flavor a dish. Curry sold for the American market is not as hot.

Curries are wonderful for using up leftovers; any meat may be substituted for the lamb.

1 pound boneless lamb shoulder
½ cup oil
2 medium onions, diced
2 small apples, diced
1 to 2 teaspoons curry powder
½ teaspoon salt
¼ teaspoon pepper
¼ teaspoon cinnamon
1 cup bouillon

Cut meat into cubes and brown in oil. Set meat aside.

Add onions and apples to oil and cook over low heat until both are very soft. Add curry powder, salt, pepper, and cinnamon. Mix well. Add bouillon and stir while heating to a boil. Reduce heat.

Add meat, cover, and simmer over a low heat until tender. This should take about 30 minutes.

Calories per 3-ounce serving: 240

Makes 6 servings

Veal Stew

If you substitute veal for beef in this traditional German dish, you will reduce the number of calories considerably. Instead of altering the flavor of the stew, the veal will improve it.

1 pound lean veal cut into 1-inch cubes
1 cup chicken or beef broth
1 small onion into which two cloves have been stuck
1 bay leaf
1 teaspoon salt
1 small lemon slice

1 teaspoon vinegar
1 tablespoon cornstarch
2 tablespoons water

Heat broth with onion, bay leaf, salt, lemon, and vinegar. Strain the liquid and add veal. Simmer veal until tender (about 1 to 1½ hours). Remove veal and keep hot in oven.

Mix cornstarch with water. Bring broth to a boil and add water and cornstarch mixture, stirring constantly. Cook until thickened and clear. Add veal and heat. Garnish with chopped parsley.

Calories per 3-ounce serving: 250

Makes 6 servings

Poached Fish

If you can interest your family in fish, this is one of the best ways to prepare it. Poaching prevents the drying out, which makes so many people turn away from fish.

Cod, halibut, or haddock can be used for this recipe.

1 pound fish fillets, cod, halibut, or haddock (frozen or fresh)
1 cup water
1 teaspoon salt
1 tablespoon lemon juice
4 peppercorns
½ small onion, sliced
1 bay leaf
1 teaspoon vinegar

Simmer all ingredients—except the fish—together for five minutes. Strain stock and pour over fish.

Simmer until fish has lost its translucency. Do not allow stock to come to a boil.

Calories per 3-ounce serving: 135

Makes 3 to 4 servings

Salmon Croquettes

Salmon is another fish that allows the diet cook to keep up the protein level but reduce the calories at the supper table. These croquettes are a main dish which is just as filling as a steak.

2 cups cooked rice, cooled
1 can (6½ to 7 ounces) flaked salmon
2 teaspoons minced parsley
1 egg, separated
6 stuffed olives
2 tablespoons water
½ cup dry bread crumbs
1-inch oil in deep fry pan

Combine rice, salmon, parsley, and egg yolk. Shape into six oval croquettes, placing a stuffed olive inside each one.

Mix the egg white and water. Dip croquettes into this mixture, drain, and then coat with bread crumbs. Let coating dry.

Fry in oil heated to 375°F for 2 to 3 minutes, until golden brown. Drain on paper towels. To serve, arrange on a hot platter.

Calories per croquette: 250
Makes 6 portions

Peach Upside-Down Cake

Desserts for the dieting child are a problem that can never be laid completely to rest. Fresh or canned fruit served in ice water instead of syrup are still my favorite desserts. But for special occasions or for times when you think a sweet tooth needs to be satisfied, this is an excellent recipe.

2 egg whites
¾ cup sugar
1 cup and 2 tablespoons flour
1 teaspoon baking powder
1 tablespoon salt
2½ tablespoons oil
½ cup buttermilk
1½ teaspoons vanilla

Heat oven to 350°F. Oil lightly and flour one 9-inch-layer cake pan or a medium-size, oven-resistant skillet.

Beat egg whites until frothy. Gradually beat in ½ cup sugar. Continue beating until the meringue is stiff and glossy. Sift remaining sugar, flour, baking powder, and salt into another bowl. Add oil, buttermilk, and vanilla. Stir until smooth. Fold in meringue.

Topping

2 tablespoons oil
2 tablespoons brown sugar
6 peach halves

Mix oil and brown sugar and spread over bottom of cake pan or skillet.

Cut peach halves into even crescents and place them in a petal design at the bottom of the pan. Pour in the batter and bake the cake for 35 minutes, or until it tests done.

Calories per slice: 120

Makes 16 pieces

12

Why Exercise?

Dieting is half the battle; the other half is exercise. Your child will quickly discover that losing weight alone will not give him the strong, vigorous body about which he's been dreaming. Flabby arms, heavy thighs, and the old rolltop stomach will still remain. The only way you can turn a fat, soft body into a strong, healthy body is exercise.

In theory, a person drops one dress or suit size for every ten pounds of weight he loses. But in practice, some of my campers shrink four sizes in one summer even though they have lost only twenty-five pounds. The secret is exercise. The youngsters not only dropped pounds, they also redistributed the weight that remained and tightened their figures.

Overweight children often have a built-in resistance to exercise. They don't like to move fast because they weigh so much. Yet sitting around thinking about more food makes them even fatter, and, as a consequence, they feel even less like exerting themselves.

When they go on a diet, overweight children often resist the idea that exercise is as necessary to losing weight as is the cutting down of calories. I wish I had a nickel for every summer-camp lawyer who has argued that it takes twenty minutes of walking to burn off the calories from one slice of bread, and thirty minutes to work off the calories from two pats of butter. Many even quote some eminent diet authority! They suggest that I cut down the amount of food I serve and stop trying to get them to exercise and move faster all the time.

I have to tell them that dieting isn't selective, and that they can't control what part of their body loses the pounds. It is true that if they don't exercise, they can still lose weight by dieting. But by summer's end they'll be small and flabby instead of big and flabby.

Furthermore, the campers often argue that exercise will increase their appetites. Actually, people who exercise more eat *less* than people who do nothing all day. This has been proven in scientific tests, but my campers don't believe it until they have exercised vigorously for a couple of weeks. Then they find that they are so interested in the life around them that they are too busy to worry about their stomachs. They come to meals feeling stronger and more vigorous, instead of experiencing that old ravenous feeling that used to come from doing nothing but worry about food all the time.

If your child seems sluggish about exercise and remains skeptical about physical activity as an aid to losing weight, point out that for every 3,500 calories burned up in physical activity, he will lose one pound of body fat. Show him this chart:

Activity	*Calories Used Per Hour*
Sitting down	35
Standing still	100
Walking slowly	140
Washing and dressing	160
Volleyball	210
Cleaning house	230
Ironing	260
Rapid walking	300
Ice skating	350
Ping-Pong	350

Activity	*Calories Used Per Hour*
Bicycling	400
Dancing	500
Tennis	500
Horseback riding	500
Skiing	600
Swimming	750
Jogging	800 to 900!

Using a pencil and paper, show your child what would happen if he went horseback riding for an hour just twice a week. He'd burn up 52,000 calories in one year. At 3,500 calories per pound, that would come to nearly 15 pounds of weight lost, as well as tightening and strengthening his stomach, leg, and thigh muscles.

Of course, nothing ever works out in real life with quite such mathematical exactness. But this is a good indication of what exercise could do for your child if he sticks to it faithfully.

Exercise in itself won't help him lose much weight. But without it, his diet program won't be as effective.

Please start slowly. If your child is used to a sedentary life, you can overtax his system if you plunge him too quickly into a strenuous program of physical exercise. In addition to doing him physical harm, it can discourage him from wanting to exercise again. Even if he manages to survive a sudden emphasis on physical activity in his life, he will probably find that he can't perform at sports as well as his peers. And despite the sympathy of other youngsters, his inability to perform might prove too jarring to his self-image. As a result, he may resist any attempts to exercise again.

Go slowly. Introduce the *idea* of exercise first, pointing out its benefits, then find the activities he likes and encourage him to participate. If he's not naturally athletic or aggressive, convince him to try activities in which he can measure his progress against himself.

For example, swimming, ice skating, jogging, horseback riding, and even skiing are activities which one does essentially alone. There are no established standards of performance for the child to meet. And if others do not think he is a very good rider or skier, he can measure his performance against his own capabilities six months earlier and feel that he has made great progress.

Your child will get about five hours of light activity a day —doing classwork, watching television, talking on the telephone. In addition, he can spend eight hours involved in activities that could be classified as light exercise, such as walking, typing, and cleaning his room. But the remaining three hours should be devoted to more energetic activity before he gets his eight hours' sleep.

In the category of more vigorous physical activity are gymnastics, team sports, calisthenics, jogging, and swimming. Three hours a day will seem like a long time to your child—and to you—to be spent in such physical activity. But if it's interspersed throughout the day, it shouldn't prove too demanding. For instance, a youngster might start his day with some calisthenics and a brief run around the block. On a school day when there is a gym class, he should be able to allot an hour to more demanding physical activity. Instead of dawdling to and from school, he can walk vigorously or ride a bicycle. Then an hour or an hour and a half of lively physical activity after school, and your child will have met his daily need for physical exercise.

Some schools have a well-developed extracurricular sports program which allows children who are not good athletes to participate at their level of competence. But there are still systems in which the school athletic program is oriented to Big Team sports and is based upon a win-at-any-cost philosophy. Unfortunately, the overweight child is neglected in such situations.

In these cases, it is the parents' responsibility to find an activity for their child. In most communities, there is a YMCA or YMHA or a community center that runs a sports program. But again, the overweight child may feel diffident about joining; he may be afraid of exposing himself to ridicule or damaging his self-image. If this is so, enroll the youngster in private lessons. I know they can be expensive initially, but if they help your child gain a lifelong interest in a physical activity, it is money well invested.

For girls, dance and yoga classes are still popular and very healthy. They not only provide good exercise but they also help develop good posture and gracefulness.

For boys, I used to recommend golf and tennis lessons but today, I find more of them interested in karate and other forms of self-defense. (Many girls are interested as well.)

Although I am not in favor of violent behavior of any kind, I believe that karate lessons can prove very beneficial from the standpoints of exercise and physical discipline. Furthermore, a reputable karate teacher will teach the youngsters not to misuse the skills they develop.

The most significant gain from karate is the self-confidence which I have seen develop in youngsters who used to be afraid of their own shadows.

If you start to discuss exercise with your son or daughter, and they confess that they have always had a secret yen to become a black-belt karate expert, don't throw up your hands in despair. Seek out a reputable karate club, explain your child's special problems, and enroll your child in a suitable class. You will be helping him in several ways.

The most important part of exercise is consistency. Encourage your child to try new physical activities, but make sure he finally sticks with one, or even better, two activities so that he can vary them with the seasons. Starting one form of physical exercise and then dropping it a couple of weeks later serves no constructive purpose.

13

Posture and Figure Exercises

Exercise, like everything else involved in losing weight, begins at home. If your child can develop a good set of exercises which he will do faithfully in his room, it will not only help him shape up as he loses weight through dieting, but it will give him a headstart in developing the skills he wants to show off to others.

Take a good look at your child one morning when he least expects it. How he stands and how he moves are good indications of what he thinks of himself. If he has been overweight for a long time, chances are he walks with his shoulders hunched over and stares at the floor as if he were wishing there were some way he could sink through it and be freed of all his troubles.

If you can get him to stand up straight, you'll find that he looks better and even a bit thinner. And this, of course, will greatly improve his state of mind. Have your child stand against a wall, feet about three inches from it. If his posture is perfect, his head, shoulders, and buttocks will be touching the wall and the small of his back won't be more than a hand's thickness away.

Then have him stand against a full-length mirror and divide his profile with an imaginary—or real—plumb line, from the top of his head to his feet. It should divide him in half at the shoulder, the hip, the knee, and the anklebone. If it doesn't, and if he leaves embarrassing gaps when standing against the wall, then it's time to start these posture- and figure-improving exercises.

1. With feet about two inches from the base of a wall, stand with the whole spine touching the wall, arms straight at sides, head and shoulders back. Slowly bend the knees and slide down the wall to a sitting position. Hold this position for a count of five. Then push the body up the wall with every part of the spine touching it. Tense and squeeze the buttocks, keeping the hips tucked under and pressing the small of the back to the wall.

In the beginning, repeat this exercise four times daily and gradually increase it to twenty times a day.

2. Sit against the wall with legs crossed, arms against the wall and all vertebrae touching it. Slide arms up until straight above your head. Repeat ten times.

3. Lie on the floor with arms overhead, knees bent, feet flat on the floor. Pull in abdomen so that the small of the back presses against the floor, hold this position, and then relax. Repeat ten times.

4. Lie on the floor with knees bent, feet flat, and arms bent at the elbows. Pull in the abdomen while straightening arms and legs. Count to ten and then relax. Repeat ten times.

Children begin calisthenics with vigor and purpose, but then boredom sets in from doing the same set of exercises every morning. However, I have found that if the youngsters develop an interest in a particular sport—tennis and skiing are particularly popular—they will often undertake a daily set of exercises designed to improve their skill in it.

Calisthenics are excellent for strengthening and toning up the body. A youngster should be able to do the exercises in his room, but any space, six by six feet will do. If the exercise area is not carpeted, provide him with thick beach towels or a rubber mat.

Here are some calisthenic exercises for children who are trying to lose weight.

1. Stand with your feet apart, holding a towel in front of you. Pulling hard on the ends of the towel, raise it slowly until your arms are straight over your head. Bending your elbows slightly, lower your arms and then lower towel behind your back. Relax and return to original position. Repeat exercise three times.

2. Stand with your feet apart and hold a towel over your head. Keeping your arms straight, bend to the left as far as you can, then to the right as far as you can. Repeat five times, alternating sides.

3. Stand with your feet apart, holding a towel over your head. Keeping your arms straight, bend and touch your left hand to your right foot. Straighten up slowly, then touch your right hand to your left foot. Repeat five times, alternating sides.

One of the best places to do exercises is in the bath. A child has absolute privacy, and he is very much aware of his excess weight. The sight of the bulges and rolls often inspires him to do something about it immediately.

The following simple exercises for the tub can be surprisingly effective.

1. Sit up in the bath, back straight and arms relaxed in the water. Slowly roll head to the right, back to the left, and down in the front. Repeat twice, then practice the same motions to the right twice.

2. Sit up straight, arms relaxed at your sides. Hunch your shoulders forward, up, back, and down. The effect should be a slow rolling of the shoulders. Repeat the roll three times forward and three times backward.

3. Lie back in the tub and slowly pull in your stomach muscles. Hold them in for a count of ten and then relax. Repeat five times.

4. Lie back in the tub and keep your right leg straight as you slowly bend your left leg and swing it over your right, trying to touch the bottom of the tub with your left knee. Then keep your left leg straight and try to touch the bottom of the tub with your right knee. (This is an excellent exercise for reducing hips.) Repeat five times, alternating sides.

14

The Beautiboot—Secret Weapon Exerciser

My secret weapon in the war on fat is the beautiboot, which I invented and hold a U.S. government patent on. I believe it is the best way to reduce legs and thighs and develop a good figure.

Years ago while working with figure skaters, I began to notice that no matter how bad a skater's figure might be, she had beautiful legs. The answer, of course, was the skates. The skaters were performing difficult exercises with weights attached to their feet.

When I started to work with overweight children, I applied the lessons I had learned from the figure skaters and the result was the beautiboot.

One of my campers read in *Vogue* magazine that Princess Pignatelli, the fashion designer, was trying to reduce her thighs by exercising with a towel stuffed with bullets tied to her feet. My camper wrote the editor of *Vogue* about the Camp Stanley beautiboot, and the editor called me to find out about it. I told her about the beautiboot, and she asked me to send a pair to the princess. I did, and the princess sent me a grateful letter in reply.

Homemade beautiboots are simple to make. All you need are four pounds of dried beans or peas, two yards of one-inch-wide ribbon or tape, and two 18-inch square measures of heavy cloth—towels or napkins will do.

For each beautiboot:

1. Place two pounds of peas or beans, either two 1-pound packages or two pounds in a strong plastic bag, at an angle in the center of the cloth.

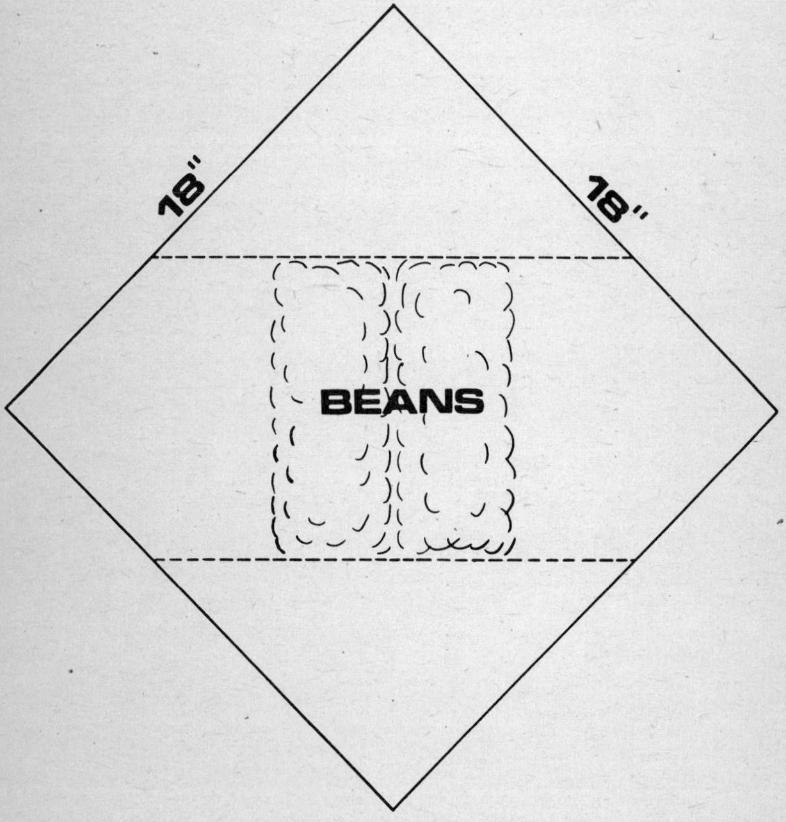

2. Fold the opposite corners of the napkin over the beans to the width of the beans. Then stitch through the cloth along

the length of the package and sew down the flap so that the beans will not slide out. Now you have a small "pillow" stuffed with beans.

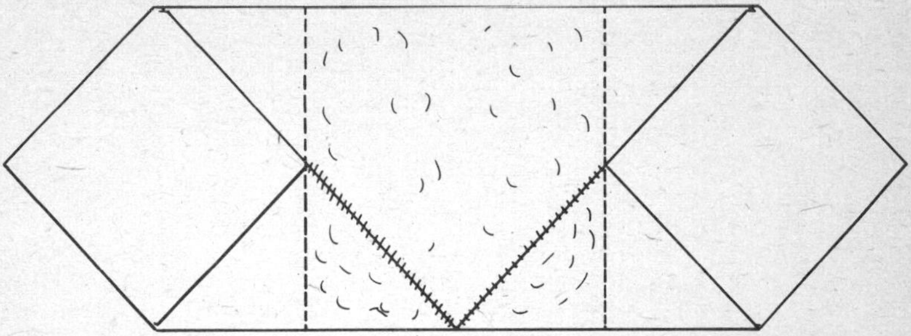

3. Fold the other corners of the cloth over the pillow so that the tips touch. Once again, stitch along the sides of the pillow for extra strength.

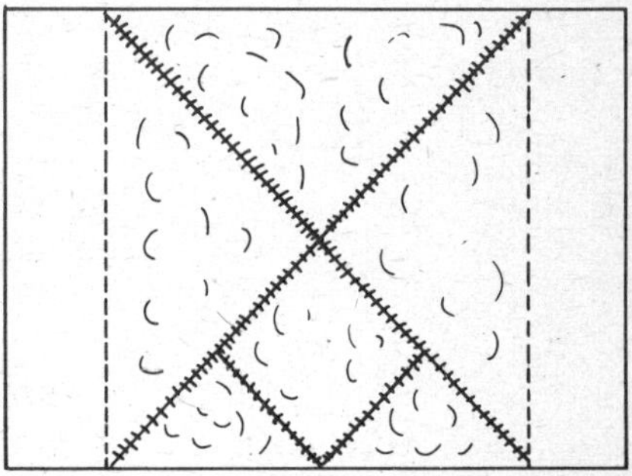

4. Turn over the pillow so that the open part faces down, and center a one-yard length of ribbon or tape across the width of the pillow. Using strong thread, attach the ribbon to the pillow and to the material at the sides. The beautiboot is finished.

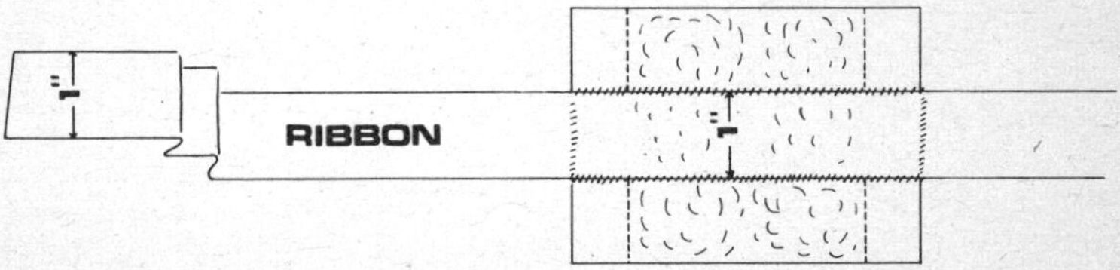

When you have made two beautiboots, place the pillows under your feet and tie the beautiboots on as you would sandals. With the ribbons tied securely about your ankles, you are ready to begin exercising. Ten minutes of exercise with these boots will equal thirty minutes of exercise without them. But before you begin, let me give you three tips on using the boots.

1. Always point your heels instead of your toes. Your toes will be pointing straight up, which is the best position for exercise.

2. Lift only one leg at a time. Don't try lifting both legs off the floor together until you're in good condition and you're accustomed to using the beautiboot.

3. Don't stand in the boots, they are for exercise only.

Now to the exercises.

For the Thighs

Lie on your side with your arm under your head. (You can brace yourself with your other hand.) Slowly raise your leg as high as possible and hold it there for a count of ten. Relax and bring your leg down slowly. Repeat the exercise ten times on each side.

At first, it won't seem as if the two-pound weight in the beautiboot is having much effect. But, believe me, it's working for you.

For the Chest and Back

Lie on your back with your arms over your head, and legs bent slightly. Press the heels of your beautiboots firmly against the floor. Slowly lift your body to a sitting position, and fold your arms in front of you. Hold this position for a count of ten, then lie down again.

Remember to exhale when you are coming to a sitting position and to inhale when you are going down. Try to do this exercise ten times, but work up to that gradually.

For Thighs and Midriff

Lie on your back with your arms outstretched. Slowly raise your right leg, and then your left leg until your knees are touching the chest. Slowly swing your legs from side to side, pulling your midriff in. Try to do the exercise ten times, working up to that number gradually.

15

Tips for Dieting Insurance

By now I hope you realize that my weight-reduction system is really a combination of love, common sense, and painstaking care.

Once you have got into the habit of counting calories when you cook, and you have got your child into the habit of seeking out healthy foods instead of fattening ones, you're on your way. It's a matter of sticking to your resolve and making good food habits a vital part of your life.

In this final chapter, you will find some practical tips for making weight reduction and control work.

At Home

(1) Weigh your child each morning before breakfast and mark the weight on a calendar.

(2) Hang a mirror over the refrigerator.

(3) Give your child a holiday now and then. Let him gorge

himself. You can reduce his calorie intake slightly for a few days (his feasting will probably show up on the scale) until his weight comes down again.

(4) Get up ten minutes earlier and do calisthenics with your children every day.

(5) Teach your children, not just the overweight ones, how to cook.

(6) Teach your daughter to sew or enroll in a sewing class with her. The girl who can save money by making her own clothes is ahead of the game, and studying patterns and cutting cloth will give the fat girl a new sense of her body's shape.

(7) Encourage your children to redecorate their rooms alone. Provide the tools—hammer, saw, nails, wallpaper, and paint. When you're starting a weight-control program, it's a great morale booster to change your environment in some way at the same time. And redecorating a room is a fine, calorie-burning exercise.

(8) Keep a plastic bag of celery, carrot sticks, or fruit in the refrigerator for those moments when not even the mirror image of fat can deter your overweight child from seeking a snack.

(9) Give your child a large glass of water or a light soup at the beginning of a meal. These are harmless appetite quenchers, and the youngster will be less tempted to eat hearty portions of the main course and dessert.

(10) If your whole family needs to lose weight, then set a collective goal, say 100 pounds for four people. When the great day comes and everybody lines up for your weekly weigh-in and you discover that the family, as a group, has lost 100 pounds, celebrate. Buy something everyone in the family has always wanted, or go out for a night on the town.

This formula avoids the kind of comparison and competitiveness that can occur when two or more people in one family are trying to lose weight. It also provides a goal for your dieting child—or children.

Outside the Home

(1) Organize a club for children who are trying to lose weight. There are many national groups that provide formats for organizing adult weight-reduction clubs, and you can either adapt one of these to suit your childrens' needs, or organize it yourself. Youngsters can derive great comfort and moral strength from discussing their mutual problems.

(2) Organize a club for mothers whose children are on diets. You, too, can benefit from discussion of similar problems.

(3) Organize a jogging or a bicycle club. Either activity will help burn up calories.

(4) Encourage your child to "pair up" with a child who is undertaking a similar weight-reduction program. They can do exercises together and telephone one another whenever the urge to nibble something fattening arises.

(5) Give your child an orange or an apple to eat on the way home from school.

(6) Ask a friendly doctor for a note saying your child is on a diet and shouldn't be given starchy foods in the school cafeteria.

(7) If you know a *really* friendly doctor, have him write a note saying your child is "allergic" to fattening foods.

(8) Encourage your child to find a new route to and from school. If he doesn't pass the old familiar candy store, chances are he won't be tempted to buy a sweet snack.

(9) Arrange a set of aptitude tests through your school, YMCA, or community center. Discovering your child's hidden talents and encouraging him to develop them is one of the best ways I know to take his mind off food.

(10) Ask your doctor or school guidance counselor for the name of someone in your neighborhood who has lost weight. Then arrange a meeting with your child. After you have made the introduction, fade out of sight. Curiosity and human nature will do the rest.

Eating Out

(1) Carry a few packets of saccharin with you. Most restaurants now stock saccharin as a matter of course, but it is a good idea to have some with you.

(2) If you're looking for a place to eat, try a good Chinese restaurant. The sauces are less fattening than those served in American- or European-style restaurants. If your child stays clear of shrimp rolls and fried noodles and restricts himself to one scoop of boiled rice with his food, he'll be fine.

(3) Second choice should be a seafood restaurant.

(4) A good, standard, American restaurant should be your last choice. But if this is where preference or circumstances lead you, keep your calorie counter in mind. Look for shrimp cocktails, bouillon, and boiled meat.

(5) If your child is a teen-ager, chances are he's not going to take you along to drive-in restaurants. Try to convince him that the best food at a drive-in is a chicken salad sandwich and a diet drink. If he feels embarrassed about ordering chicken salad in front of his friends, suggest that he order a hot dog, throw away the roll, and eat it slowly.

(6) At a wedding reception or one of those affairs at which waiters march around with trays full of goodies, teach your child to reach for cheese squares, small frankfurters, or shrimps. Or even better, get him to reach for melon balls.

(7) When going on a car trip, carry fruit and a thermos full of juice to still any hunger pangs.

(8) On a fishing trip, pack some cans of tuna and salmon. If your child doesn't catch anything, he can still enjoy some low-calorie fish meals.

(9) On a long car trip, do not travel too far between stops. And, when you stop, try to pick a place that will have a reasonable selection of food.

(10) When traveling, avoid American-plan hotels that include meals in the price of the room. Stick to European-plan hotels that allow your child to choose the food he wants.

Well, I've given you the basic information, the tools to do the job. From now on, helping your child lose weight is your responsibility. I hope that you have as much success with your child as I have had with the girls and boys at Camp Stanley and Camp Tahoe.

About the Author

Gussie Mason is a leading nutritionist and director of Camp Stanley and Camp Tahoe, two weight-reducing camps in New York's Catskill Mountains. She founded the camps fifteen years ago to help unhappy and overweight girls and boys shed pounds and learn to live active, healthy lives.

Overweight herself as a teenager, Mrs. Mason recognizes the emotional problems that can lead to and maintain obesity in youngsters. She says, "If there had only been a Camp Stanley when I was a young girl, I would have been spared all those years of misery." Today, a trim size 10 and grandmother of five, Mrs. Mason receives letters of gratitude from children and their parents across the country attesting to the phenomenal success of her carefully planned camp regimen and her ability to "reach" the campers. In *HELP YOUR CHILD LOSE WEIGHT And Keep It Off*, Gussie Mason makes her nonmedical reducing program for children available to parents everywhere.

Mrs. Mason has appeared on such television programs as "Girl Talk" and "To Tell The Truth." A National Film Board of Canada film "A Matter of Fat," narrated by movie and television star Lorne Greene, features many scenes taken at Camps Stanley and Tahoe.